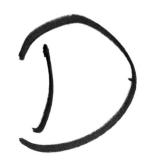

D1025116

My Tummy Hurts

A Complete Guide to
Understanding and Treating
Your Child's Stomachaches

Joseph Levy, M.D.

FIRESIDE
Rockefeller Center
1230 Avenue of the Americas
New York, NY 10020

For information regarding special discounts for bulk purchases,
please contact Simon & Schuster Special Sales at
1-800-456-6798 or business@simonandschuster.com.

Book design by William Ruoto

Manufactured in the United States of America

1   3   5   7   9   10   8   6   4   2

Library of Congress Cataloging-in-Publication Data
Levy, Joseph.
My tummy hurts : a complete guide to understanding and treating your
child's stomachaches / Joseph Levy.
p.   cm.
Includes index.
1. Pediatric gastroenterology—Popular works. I. Title.
RJ446.L478 2004
618.92'33—dc22
2003070448

ISBN 0-7432-3606-8

Contents

Acknowledgments

This book is the result of decades of experience with thousands of patients and their parents. I am grateful to so many for sharing their observations and showing me the constructive and creative ways in which a family can respond to the daily challenge of such a deceptively simple complaint as "my tummy hurts."

The project began in a series of conversations with the writer Ian Jackman, and it grew with his transcription of our morning talks. A few friends and parents deserve special mention here for their support and willingness to review parts of the manuscript in its early stages: Jacky Beshar, for her energizing and unwavering support; Renee Khatami, who over the years has been the model of a dedicated and committed parent; Debra Mandelbaum, a marvelous sounding board and believer in my clinical work; Helen Morris, an intellectual powerhouse and opener of wide horizons; Sasha Wade, for her sensitivity, sensibility, and common sense; and Diane Volk, for her scalpel-sharp wit, constructive review of the manuscript, and contagious love of music. Last, but not least, to my friend and talented illustrator Horacio Madinaveitia: my thanks for his assistance and good humor.

Over the years, I have had the privilege of working with dedicated and compassionate colleagues who have shared generously their own experiences and wise insights. To my friend and fellow pediatric gastroenterologist, Dr. Robert Issenman, of McMaster University, Ontario, Canada, my warmest thanks for providing valuable comments. To Susan Brodlie, nutritionist par excellence at the Children's Hospital of New York Presbyterian, many thanks for her expert advice and ongoing guidance. To Dr. Walter Berdon, Professor of Radiology, Columbia University College of Physicians and Surgeons, thanks for his constant encouragement and support, not to mention his enduring and contagious love of sailing.

But when all is said and done, my greatest debt of gratitude is to my family. My parents, Alberto and Clemen Levy, have always nurtured my curiosity and love of life. My children, Nomi and Berti, have been a constant source of insight, at first by their very existence and development, and now by their maturity and perceptiveness. Their empathy for my patients, their keen ear for the language, and their involvement in this project have provided delight and illumination.

Finally, yet first and foremost, no words can adequately express my appreciation for my partner in life and on this project: my wife, Valery. She has been a source of strength and support for more than thirty-five years, and throughout my career. It is with the deepest love that I dedicate this book to her.

Introduction

Stomachaches rank second only to upper-respiratory infections as a reason for nonroutine visits to the doctor. A child's familiar complaint of "my tummy hurts" is one that a parent cannot ignore. It can conjure up your worst fears: appendicitis? food poisoning? worms? Are you overreacting? It could be just too much ice cream or Monday-morning school aversion.

Most parents feel insecure about appraising their child's symptoms and evaluating the degree of discomfort: all they can see is that their child is in pain. *My Tummy Hurts* will provide parents and caregivers with a guide to the puzzling and often frightening topic of stomachaches. It will enhance your ability to ask the right questions and identify the problems, as well as offer practical advice to provide a clearer analysis of the problem. It will show how to manage common problems and how to recognize the important factors that make the difference between benign forms of pain and those requiring immediate or urgent medical attention.

Taking care of children is a partnership between the caregiver and the health care provider. The better the communication between them, the better the care will be. Much of what physicians use to reach a diagnosis is based on having an accurate history of the problem, knowing the sequence of events, and assessing the child's response. It *is* all in the details. As facts and details—and test results, if appropriate—accumulate, the diagnosis becomes apparent.

And so, after over twenty years of experience as a pediatric gastroenterologist, I have spent many hours fielding questions from parents, moving them along to a better understanding of their child's problem, and giving them a solid handle on how things work. With a clearer picture of how the intestine works and why it hurts, parents become more confident about their own instincts and observations.

With this philosophy in mind, the organization of part I of *My Tummy Hurts* was developed to provide a general foundation on how the digestive system works and how to maintain good health through proper nutrition. It starts with chapter 1, "The Digestive System and How It Works," which introduces the components of the gastrointestinal tract and the interrelationships among them. In chapter 2, "Nutrition: What to Eat, When to Eat, and How Much to Eat," provides commonsense advice on building good eating habits and making mealtimes less stressful. The United States Department of Agriculture's New Food Pyramid is also presented, and the reasons for changes to the recommendations of previous models are explained.

In part II, "Why Does the Tummy Hurt? Pinpointing Pain," I explore the reasons for stomachache pain and what to look for when a child complains. When parents have the tools to more accurately describe the character, location, and timing of the pain, they will be better able to assist in figuring out what is wrong. The role of stress and the interaction between the "brain in the gut" and our conscious awareness of the pain is also reviewed, and new strategies are provided to conquer and successfully cope with chronic pain. I conclude part II with chapter 5's description of diagnostic tests that help investigate digestive problems ("Digestive Detective: Diagnostic Gastrointestinal Tests"). There you will find such practical information as descriptions of various common tests, the duration of each, why it is performed, what preparation is needed, and what you can tell your child about it.

In part III, "The Most Common Gastrointestinal Disorders," I describe those frequently encountered conditions for which a general understanding will enhance parents' ability to recognize and manage the problems more effectively. Included are chapters on feeding difficulties, infantile colic, acid reflux, gas, lactose intolerance, diarrhea, and constipation. Each chapter briefly describes one of these conditions, how it manifests itself, what is needed to confirm the diagnosis, and what can be done to treat it effectively. These chapters need not be read sequentially— and certainly not in one sitting: they are there for you to review when needed.

Finally, part IV, "When It's More Than Just Pain," covers how to choose a pediatric gastroenterologist, as well as some of the less common conditions such as inflammatory bowel disease, celiac disease, *H. pylori* gastritis, pancreas and liver disorders, and cyclic vomiting syndrome (CVS). Although these conditions fortunately occur much less frequently than those discussed in part III, many parents whose individual circumstances dictate it will find the information useful and reliable.

Reading the book will familiarize you with many aspects of normal digestive and nutritional health and will enhance your understanding of gastrointestinal problems. Whether or not your child is suffering from any of these conditions, sooner or later, this information will come in handy and will allow you to manage your child's complaints with self-assurance.

I

Knowledge Is Power

CHAPTER 1

The Digestive System
and How It Works

When it comes to your child's health, knowledge really is power. Being an informed parent will give you clearer insight into what is causing your child's chronic reflux, persistent diarrhea, or feeding difficulty. You will know exactly what to look for and how to better describe what you have observed the next time you call up or visit the doctor's office. Having a common vocabulary improves communication between you and your doctor and will help you become a genuine partner in your child's treatment.

This discussion of the digestive system will not only introduce this vocabulary but will also fill the gaps you may have in your understanding about how the body works. What is the role of bacteria in the colon? How do we digest milk? What does the pancreas do? Where is it located? Such questions and more will be addressed: the following description of the digestive system provides a picture of how it works under normal circumstances, as well as information you can refer back to when reading about the various conditions this book tackles in subsequent chapters.

The Digestive System

The food you give your child makes a finely orchestrated journey along a tube that begins at the mouth and ends with the anus. This tube is the major component of the gastrointestinal, or GI, system, which is known as the digestive tract, the intestinal tract, or, simply, the gut, and comprises the esophagus, stomach, and small and large intestines. The digestive organs—the liver, gallbladder, and pancreas—branch off from this tube. When a child is born, the tract will typically be ten to twelve feet long; by adulthood it is twenty to twenty-five feet long.

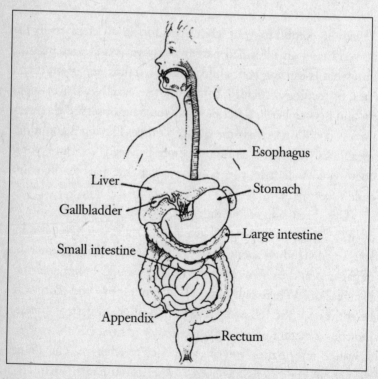

FIGURE #1   General View of the Gastrointestinal Tract

The digestive process itself gets under way even before your child is fed. He will let you know he's hungry in his own individual way. As he's getting ready to feed, his brain is sending signals that bring the digestive tract into a state of preparedness. His mouth will water because he is making saliva, and his stomach will produce acid.

THE MOUTH

When food is in the mouth, it is mixed with the saliva we make in the salivary glands located around the mouth. (See figure 2.) Saliva includes amylase and lipase, two enzymes that break down starches and fats into simpler components that our body absorbs and uses for energy and other metabolic needs. Because it works on the specific type of fat found in breast milk or formula, lipase is a particularly important enzyme for babies.

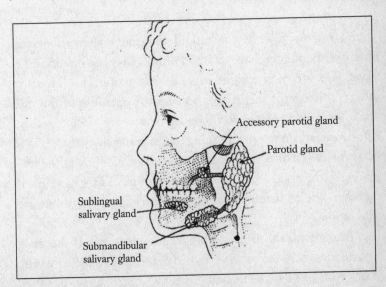

Accessory parotid gland

Parotid gland

Sublingual salivary gland

Submandibular salivary gland

FIGURE #2   The Mouth and the Salivary Glands

As a child progresses from an infant's diet of formula and/or breast milk and starts to eat more complicated foods, such as cereals, vegetables, and meats, the enzyme mix in the saliva he generates will be adapted to the particular kind of food being eaten, whether fatty, sweet, or salty. Besides carrying enzymes, saliva also helps sweep away food fragments down toward the stomach when solids are eaten. And because it contains bicarbonate, saliva works to neutralize stomach acid.

Chewing the solid food mixes it with the enzymes in the saliva and helps make the resulting mass of food, or bolus, easier to swallow, though it's not necessary to chew each mouthful a dozen times, as children might have been told. As food is chewed, the tongue pushes it toward the back of the mouth, funneling it into an area of the soft palate called the pharynx, which is the entrance to the esophagus.

SWALLOWING

The act of swallowing is a complicated one. Five or six nerves and twenty muscles have to act in unison to make sure that the food goes down the right pipe, or the esophagus. There is always a danger it might not, because the openings of the trachea, or windpipe, and the esophagus are very close together. One mechanism to prevent things from going the wrong way is that the *epiglottis*, a valve made of cartilage, closes over the trachea to stop food from entering the larynx. The gag reflex is another line of defense against food accidentally getting into the lungs.

Along with the skin and lungs, the gut is one of the main boundaries between a child's body and the outside world. Luckily, it has a sophisticated protective system against foreign bodies like bacteria and allergens. The tonsils and adenoids, found at the back of the throat, are just two parts of the immune system's protective tissue in the digestive tract.

THE ESOPHAGUS

When food is swallowed, it enters the esophagus, the tube that leads to the stomach. In a child, the esophagus is eight to ten inches long. The esophagus is made up of two layers of muscle. One layer is arranged lengthwise along the tube, the other circles it. These muscles are controlled by a system of nerves that synchronizes the muscles' contractions and expansions in such a way as to bring the food smoothly down to the stomach. The action of these sweeping waves is called *peristalsis*. (Peristalsis occurs along the whole length of the gastrointestinal tract and serves to carry food forward throughout the digestive process.)

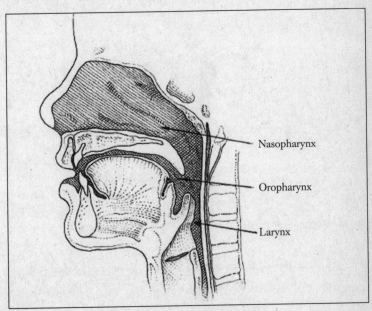

Nasopharynx

Oropharynx

Larynx

FIGURE #3   Side View of the Pharynx

At either end of the esophagus there is a *sphincter*, a ring of highly toned muscle that opens and closes to regulate the passage of food. The upper sphincter protects against food coming back up and possibly into the airway after it's been swallowed. As food reaches the end of the esophagus, the lower sphincter relaxes and allows it to enter the stomach.

A flat muscle that operates the lungs, the *diaphragm*, also divides the chest from the abdominal cavity. An opening in this flat muscle, called the *hiatus*, lets the esophagus pass through and join with the stomach. (A hiatal hernia occurs when part of the stomach slides into the chest cavity through this opening in the diaphragm.)

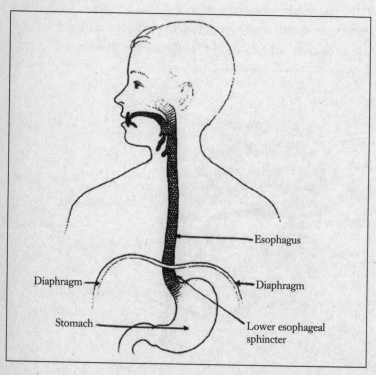

Esophagus

Diaphragm

Diaphragm

Stomach

Lower esophageal sphincter

FIGURE #4   The Esophagus

THE STOMACH

The stomach is a pear-shaped muscular bag that usually sits toward the left-hand side of the body, just below the ribs. The larger, rounder upper portion of the stomach, called the *fundus*, is able to relax and expand as it fills with food. This is why at the end of a large meal you can still find room for dessert! The narrower, tapered part of the stomach is called the *antrum*. A newborn can hold about six ounces in his stomach, an adult as much as a quart or even more—but food is not digested in the stomach—it is collected and prepared for digestion which actually happens farther along the tract, in the small intestine.

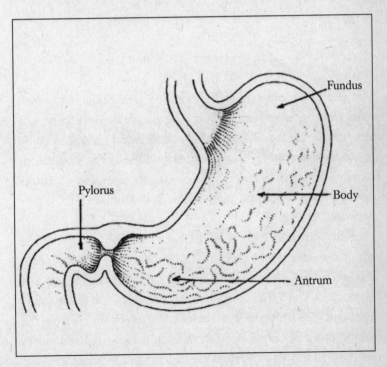

FIGURE #5   The Stomach and Its Parts

In addition to the two layers of muscle it shares with the rest of the digestive tract, the stomach has a third layer of fibers that crisscrosses the other two. This enables the antrum to move back and forth under the control of the stomach's own nervous system, churning and grinding the stomach's contents as they are combined with stomach acid and digestive enzymes.

The acid found in our stomachs is extremely powerful, so much so that it would eat away the stomach wall were the wall not protected by a special mucus. This acid has to be strong, though, because when we eat, we also take in a lot of potentially harmful yeasts and bacteria, and stomach acid is very effective at killing most of these before they leave the stomach.

How Digestion Works

Acid and enzymes in the mouth and stomach combine to break down the nutrients in our food—carbohydrates, proteins, and fats—into smaller particles that can be digested and absorbed by the small intestine. By the time the food leaves the stomach, it has been reduced to pieces one or two thousandths of a millimeter in size and mixed into a liquid with stomach acid, digestive juices, and saliva.

This liquidized food is released into the *duodenum*, the first part of the intestine, through the pyloric channel. (*Pyloros* means "gatekeeper" in Greek, a perfect description of the valve function of the muscle.) The pylorus releases only a small portion of the stomach's content at a time, as it is controlled in part by signals from the brain initiated by chemicals in the food in the stomach and movement and pressure in the stomach. A full adult stomach can take two or three hours to empty completely into the small intestine.

THE SMALL INTESTINE

The small intestine, which is also known as the small bowel and leads to the large intestine, or colon, comprises three sections: the previously mentioned duodenum, the *jejunum,* and the *ileum.* In a full-term infant, the small intestine's length is about twelve feet, while in an adult, it can be twenty feet long or more! Digestion begins in the duodenum and, under normal circumstances, most of the process is completed in the first three or four feet of intestine. The additional length provides extra surface to complete the process and serves as a backup system.

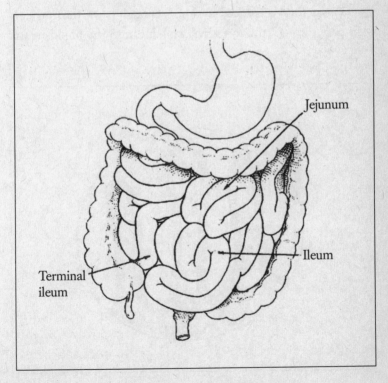

FIGURE #6   The Small Intestine

Amazingly, the intestine can detect what kind of food is present and release the appropriate hormones into the bloodstream in order to handle them properly. Hormones are chemicals that are carried by the bloodstream and have very specific functions: the hormone *gastrin*, for example, stimulates acid production, while *secretin* makes the pancreas produce digestive juices. Hormones also affect our appetite. *Ghrelin*, which was discovered quite recently, is released when there is no food in the stomach and makes us feel hungry. *Cholecystokinin* (CCK), on the other hand, has two functions: it tells the gallbladder to contract and squeeze out the bile we need to absorb fatty foods, and it tells us when we are full.

When food is reduced to simple enough parts, the nutrients can pass through the intestinal wall and into the bloodstream.

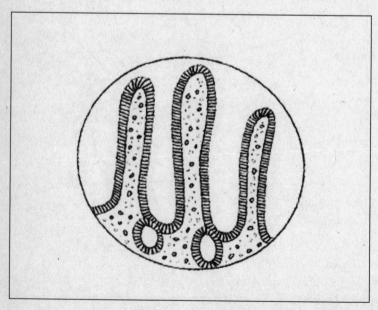

FIGURE #7   The Intestinal Villi

The intestinal wall is not smooth: it is actually covered with *villi*, tiny projections that greatly increase the surface area available for absorption. It has been estimated that the inner surface of the intestine is equivalent to the surface area of a tennis court.

Once the small intestine has done its job, all the nutrients have been extracted from food. What remains is a liquid made up of water, excess saliva, digestive juices, mineral salts, and indigestible plant fibers. Fiber is an indigestible sugar and it provides the bulk in stool.

MOTILITY

Motility refers to the forward motion (propulsion) of food from the mouth right through to its expulsion from the body. Problems with motility can explain many of the common complaints associated with a tummy ache, from spitting up and vomiting to constipation and diarrhea.

For propulsion to work well, the relaxation and contraction of the intestine's muscles have to be closely synchronized. The network of nerves in charge of these coordinated actions is called the *enteric nervous system* (ENS). The ENS is a sophisticated "brain in the gut." It is the command and control center for the gut, a complex network of nerves along which constant communication is taking place within the gut as well as with the brain. This "brain in the gut" can be a contributing factor in some tummy aches.

THE PANCREAS

The pancreas, a gland that sits just behind the stomach, delivers some of the digestive juices used in the duodenum. It is about

four to five inches long in a child, eight in an adult, and manufactures the enzymes needed to break down fat, protein, and
starches in the intestine. Its second job is to make the hormones
insulin and glucagon, which regulate our blood sugar levels.
Some of the bicarbonate that helps neutralize stomach acid is
also produced in the pancreas.

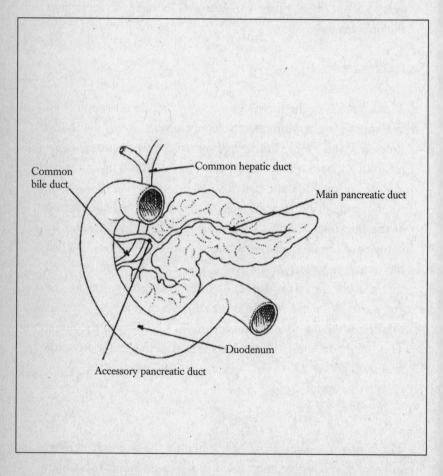

FIGURE #8   The Pancreas and Surrounding Organs

THE GALLBLADDER

The gallbladder concentrates and stores bile, which is needed to break down fat in the food in the intestine. When the gallbladder gets the signal from the intestine, it contracts and releases bile. *Lecithin,* a chemical in the bile, acts as a detergent, dissolving fat in the same way a detergent works on grease when we wash dishes.

The gallbladder sits under the surface of the liver, which is the largest organ in the digestive tract and one of the most complex organs in the body. The liver is located in the right upper side of the abdomen, protected by the ribs and chest wall.

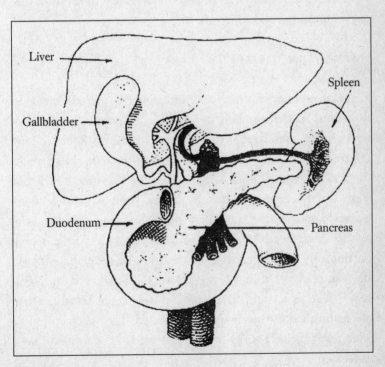

FIGURE #9   The Liver and Gallbladder

THE LIVER

The liver performs over five thousand separate metabolic tasks, which together involve an uncountable number of chemical reactions crucial to our survival. We can compensate for the loss of the gallbladder, most of the pancreas, and all of the large intestine, but we can't survive without some healthy liver.

The liver makes bile, cholesterol, and clotting factors used by the body to prevent dangerous bleeding, as well as converts glucose to glycogen, which the body stores and calls upon to help keep our sugar levels up if we are not eating properly. It can also manufacture new proteins, fats, and sugars, store iron and store the vitamins A, D, E, K, and B_{12}, and clear the body of toxins from alcohol and medications.

WASTE MANAGEMENT

Remember that once the small intestine has played its role in digestion, all that remains is a semiliquid refuse composed of water, saliva, digestive juices, salts, and fiber. This liquid follows the tract to the large intestine, also called the *colon*. In an adult, the small intestine sends about one and a half quarts of liquid waste to the large intestine each day, from which the body extracts and conserves all but a little of the fluid and reduces the rest to about five ounces of solid stool. (In a child, this is proportionately less depending on the stage of development.) As the waste moves through the colon, the water and its useful salts—such as sodium, potassium, chloride, and bicarbonate—are reabsorbed by the body and recycled. The reabsorption of water progressively turns the liquid waste into a formed bowel movement.

The colon is host to a tremendous number and variety of

bacterial flora, some five hundred species. In fact, there are ten times more bacteria in us than there are human cells! These bacteria generate important nutrients, and "good" bacteria, such as acidophilus and many others, work to forestall infection from "bad" bacteria. Acidophilus and other probiotic bacteria like it provide beneficial effects by virtue of their ability to compete against disease-producing bacteria and yeasts.

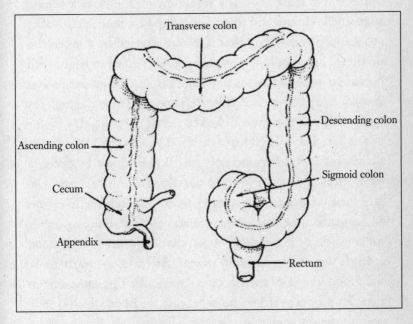

FIGURE #10   The Large Intestine (Colon)

STOOL

Normally it takes anywhere from twelve to eighteen hours for the stool to move through the colon into the rectum. The bacteria in the colon work all that time to decompose the waste, which accounts for the odor a stool can have.

One by-product of this bacterial decomposition is gas,

which can be made up of combinations of methane, carbon dioxide, hydrogen, butane, and other materials. The precise composition of the bacterial flora in the colon will vary from person to person, and this means that some people will generate more gas than others.

Babies who are on breast milk or lactose-containing formulas will not always be able to absorb all the lactose, and some of it will ferment as a result, giving the stool a slightly sour smell. Parents are often bewildered by their child's stool color and consistency. Often they are worried by a green coloration. They should not be: *every* stool is green to begin with, because it is colored with bilirubin, the same pigment present in bile. *Green stools are perfectly normal.* A green stool just means that the stool was delivered a little more quickly than it might have been. The longer the food waste stays in the colon, the darker it will become as it gets broken down by bacteria, going from green to brown to dark brown. Furthermore, certain food colorings survive the passage through the intestines and can affect the stool color, sometimes quite dramatically. As for consistency, it stands to reason that the consistency of stool changes depending on what we eat. As an infant starts to eat solid food, the stool will become more bulky. Similarly, a fiber-rich diet produces larger stools because the fiber, which is indigestible, retains water.

Once the stool has collected in the rectum, it moves down toward the first of two sphincters in the anus. The first operates automatically; the child learns to control the second one when she grows and gets potty trained. As it distends the lower sphincter, the stool causes this muscle to relax. In an infant, the waste will simply be expelled, but a child will eventually figure out when it is, or it is not, appropriate to relax the lower sphincter. If it is not the right time, she can contract the external sphincter, constrict the pelvis a little and inhibit the reflex. The stool will be forced back up into the rectum above the point where the reflex was triggered.

Bowel movement frequency can vary dramatically from person to person. A baby exclusively breast fed can go up to ten days between bowel movements, because the milk is effectively broken down and absorbed, leaving very little residue. When the stool comes and it is soft and there is no distress accompanying its passing, then a parent has nothing to worry about. Some babies will have a bowel movement when they are at the breast or on the bottle but this too is no cause for concern: we all have reflexes that encourage the large intestine to empty when food is detected in the stomach, as if the system is emptying itself and

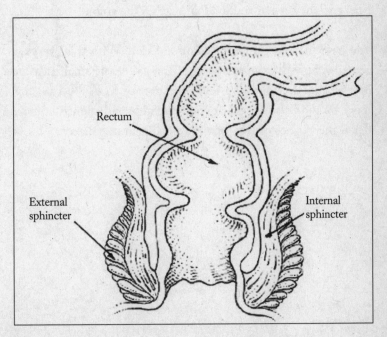

FIGURE #11   The Rectum and Its Sphincters

getting ready for the next meal. This is called the stomach-to-colon reflex, or gastrocolic reflex.

The principle behind stool frequency of breast-fed babies applies to older children as well. You might be the parent of a child who has a bowel movement only every second or third day, but as long as the child doesn't exhibit any pain or discomfort, these intervals can be acceptable.

Gastrointestinal activity and performance will also change depending on what we eat. Babies ingest only formula and milk while toddlers add simple solids. A five-year-old might have a very limited diet while an adolescent in the middle of a growth spurt will eat anything and everything in sight. The complexity of the diet plays an important role in functions such as the emptying of the stomach, food's transit time through the small intestine, and the type of residue that reaches the colon.

You have made it through the introduction! With this overview covering how the various parts of the gastrointestinal tract are involved in the ingestion and digestion of food, we can now move on to the principles of good nutrition and address in more detail the various causes for abdominal pain in children.

CHAPTER 2

Nutrition: What to Eat, When to Eat, and How Much to Eat

Chapter 1 provided an overview of the gastrointestinal (GI) tract's anatomy and briefly explained how it manages to process the complex mixture of foods we consume each day. It is a remarkable system, able to provide us with life-sustaining, and almost maintenance-free, service for decades. But sooner or later, we eat or drink something that causes trouble, and perhaps a virus infects the GI tract or a more chronic condition damages parts of it, forcing it to compensate or work at a disadvantage.

As everybody knows, nutrition is a very important element in keeping the digestive system working optimally. As the saying goes, we are what we eat, and thus what we eat, if we are not able to process it properly, will have noticeable effects on our health. Many causes of stomach pain can be directly traced to our diets; lactose intolerance and allergies to cow's milk and peanut proteins are just a few common ones. In this chapter, then, we address some of the concerns about proper nutrition in children. As a part of that discussion, we review the body's built-in wisdom and control signals, for they help us to use common sense in dealing with unexpected change, and we also examine some misconceptions that exist regarding the proper size of portions for infants and children. Finally, we provide some useful guidelines to monitor adequate growth, which usually is a good reflector of adequate nutrition in children.

Most important, this information will guide parents as to how to provide good nutrition without generating antagonism and stubbornness, force-feeding, or establishing feeding patterns that are counterproductive and unnecessary. For example, should you spend time trying to make your child eat his spinach? Well . . . no! The iron in spinach is actually very poorly absorbed. It is barely available to the body, so it is not a particularly nutritious food, although it is a reasonable source of fiber and provides some folic acid—if it's not overcooked, that is. There is really no good reason to fear that if your child doesn't eat a portion of spinach or a green vegetable every day that she's going to miss crucial nutrients. The moral of the story is that parents can be flexible yet still provide proper nutrition to their children by becoming familiar with alternative sources of essential nutrients, adjusting food choices to their child's taste preferences, and avoiding the pitfall of creating a battleground atmosphere around mealtimes.

Eating Together

Ideally, mealtime should be an occasion when the family gathers and enjoys time together. In many societies, in fact, not eating together is unthinkable, but in some families, it is often very difficult to get everyone to sit down and eat at the same time: today, a child's schedule can be as full as an adult's, and parents might return home too late from work to eat with the kids. Yet even when the family can eat together, parents, in the desire to promote good eating habits, might insist that their child eat certain foods, and this can create battlegrounds and stresses where none should exist. Mealtimes become tense, and the nurturing value of sitting around the table and sharing the day's activities gets lost.

A FAMILY THAT EATS TOGETHER . . .

Although many American families cannot eat together, the overall picture might not be totally bleak: statistics show that most young children do eat at least some meals as a family activity. Figures from the Centers for Disease Control and Prevention (CDC) show that 57 percent of young children between four and thirty-five months of age eat a midday or evening meal with family members, and another 28 percent have family meals three to six times a week. Only 3 percent never do.

I advise and encourage families to eat together as often as possible, beginning when children are very young. The effort pays off handsomely in creating cohesiveness in the family and establishing a model that can last a child's lifetime. As soon as a family can eat together, it should. Family members who encourage younger children to feed themselves at mealtimes help to promote the children's independence, socialization skills, and self-esteem.

Where to Eat

Eating together is the ideal, but in real life mealtimes with children can be difficult, for any number of reasons, and all too often, parents fall into the trap of having some kind of constant distraction going on during meals. Yet while distractions may help complete the meal with a minimum of fuss and fights, the whole idea that your child will eat better when not focused on the activity of eating should make you ask yourself why this is the case in the first place: Is the child not hungry enough at mealtimes? Is the food choice something that he truly dislikes or that made him sick in the past? Was he pulled away from a fun activity only to be buckled and constrained in the high chair?

When the problem is that a child is not hungry enough at mealtimes, it is often the result of parents following their child all over the house or playground stuffing food (or juice—overconsumption of juice can be a powerful appetite suppressant) into the child's mouth every time it happens to open. This would be funny were it not such a waste of effort and unnecessary worrying on the parents' part. Children will eat when and if they are hungry, but in trying to make sure that their children eat enough, parents who feed their children all day long ensure that their children will eat very little at mealtimes. In the process, parents will lose the benefits of structured mealtimes and a designated time and place that children associate with eating. Even worse is that they will disrupt their children's natural cycles of hunger and satiety, blurring these important body signals.

All possible causes of mealtime antagonism must be considered, however, and once problem behaviors are identified, they must be modified. Distractions should not be necessary, for not only can they be potentially harmful in the long term—the most common distraction, television, offers hypnotic images and songs that can make getting food into a child's mouth much easier, but being conditioned to eat in front of the television is a very hard habit to break and is a significant factor in overeating and subsequent obesity—but they also obscure the message that meals can be fun! For one thing, mealtimes are unique opportunities for sharing and through it, developing language and social skills in children. The joy derived by interacting with the family and others at the table and building fond memories around positive experiences is long lasting and should be encouraged.

The key, therefore, is to set up a structure early on. Food should be provided in a chosen room in the house, at regular times, for no more than forty-five to fifty minutes. Meals or snacks should not last for hours, and they certainly should not be consumed when the child is distracted or walking around. Eating in a particular room at a particular time will satisfy a child's need for structure and foster the creation of a constructive and consistent set of expectations, minimizing conflict and tension.

A designated area for eating has practical benefits as well, especially for the parents of a toddler. While learning to hold his own spoon—usually within the first two years of life—a child will inevitably make a huge mess, getting food all over himself, all over the high chair, and on the walls and floor too. So, setting aside a place in the house for meals is a must! It will simplify cleanup time and lessen frustration—and lay the groundwork for developing healthy eating habits in the coming years.

TV MANIA

The TV-Turnoff Network, an organization that encourages children and adults to watch much less television in order to promote healthier lives and communities provides two particularly telling statistics about Americans and television. The first is the average time an American child spends watching television per week: nineteen hours and forty minutes. The second is that in a four-hour block of Saturday-morning cartoons, they recorded as many as 202 ads for fast foods!

What to Eat

The commonly held belief that children left to make their own food choices will end up choosing a fairly balanced diet is probably true only *if*—and this is a big *if*—they are allowed to make their choices among healthful foods: if a child is asked to pick between a chocolate bar and a banana, he will likely choose the former. However, if the choice is between a banana or an orange, either one would be healthy. Fruits and vegetables make ideal snacks, as they are primary sources of many vitamins. (And eating the whole fruit is much healthier than drinking fruit juice!)

It is, therefore, up to parents to model and provide the right choices from early in a child's life and to do so unambiguously, consistently, positively, and enthusiastically! If the food choices presented are well balanced and nutritious, the parent can be confident that whatever the child picks will be healthy and a good source of essential vitamins.

ESSENTIAL VITAMINS AND FOODS

VITAMIN	FOODS
A	Milk, cheese, cream, fish oils
D	Butter, margarine, cream, milk, fish, cereals
E	Corn, nuts, olives, asparagus, leafy vegetables, corn oil, safflower oil
K	Cabbage, cauliflower, leafy vegetables, cereals, soybeans
B_1 (thiamine)	Meat, liver, nuts, enriched cereals, wheat germ
B_2 (riboflavin)	Milk, cheese, eggs, fish, meat, leafy vegetables, enriched grains
B_6 (pyridoxine)	Eggs, fish, milk, cereals, broccoli, cabbage, potatoes, lean meat
Niacin	Milk, cheese, cream, poultry, fish, lean meats, nuts, eggs
C	Citrus fruits, potatoes, strawberries, broccoli, leafy vegetables
Folate	Leafy vegetables

Although perhaps self-evident, it is worth repeating: if you bring healthy food home, even a picky child will be picky among good things. Problems can occur when you have the fridge filled with forbidden foods, items being saved for the bribes: "If you're good, I'll give you that." Again, one of the consequences of bad food habits can be obesity, a critical issue for our society.

VITAMINS FOUND IN SELECTED FRUITS AND VEGETABLES	
FRUIT	VITAMINS
Apple	A, C, folate, E
Banana	A, C, folate, B, niacin, pantothenic acid, E
Cantaloupe	A, C, folate, niacin
Grapes	A, C, folate, B_6
Orange	A, C, folate B_1, pantothenic acid
Strawberries	A, C, folate
VEGETABLE	VITAMINS
Avocado	A, C, B_1, B_2, niacin, folate, pantothenic acid
Broccoli	A, C, niacin, pantothenic acid, B_6
Carrots	A, C, niacin, folate, pantothenic acid, B_6
Green pepper	A, C, niacin, folate
Lima beans	Pantothenic acid, niacin, folate
Mushrooms	D, Niacin, C, pantothenic acid
Onions	C, folate
Potatoes	C, niacin, pantothenic acid, B_6, folate
Sweet potatoes	A, C, pantothenic acid, niacin, folate

HELPFUL HINTS: DEVELOPING GOOD HABITS

- Do not use the bottle as a pacifier
- Do not use food and snacks as bribes
- Do not disrupt feeding schedules
- Do not be manipulated: be consistent

The Solid-Food Stage

Transitions from the bottle, or the breast, to the cup and on to solid food are important milestones. They offer many opportunities for encouraging independence.

Weaning from exclusive bottle feedings starts when a child is around five to six months old, a time when iron requirements are best provided by enriched cereals and other solids. Introduction of solids does not follow a rigid timeline, and every pediatrician and health care practitioner has his or her own preferences. Usually cereals are introduced first, followed by yellow vegetables, green vegetables, and then fruits. Meats follow at around eight months—lamb is an excellent protein source and less allergenic than other meats or fish—and eggs, starting with cooked yolks, at around ten months. (Egg whites are not usually introduced until year one because of possible allergic reactions.) Dairy products may be safely introduced by the time your child is one year old. If there is a strong family history of allergies, or if the child has had suspicious reactions with other foods, however, the introduction of cow's milk can be postponed until eighteen months or two years. It is recommended that new foods be added gradually, testing the waters, as it were, for allergic reactions. Expose your child to new items in very small amounts—equivalent to a quarter of the portion the child could typically eat—advancing to half a portion and then to a full portion over the course of a week. This approach gives you the chance to monitor any bad reactions, such as vomiting, rashes, or diarrhea.

As solids are introduced into the diet, bottle feeding should decrease to a total of about twenty ounces a day. I often have to tell parents that although milk looks like a liquid, it is actually a homogenized solid. Its nutritional value comes from its protein, fat, and sugar (lactose), and once it is digested, the body handles it the same way it would an egg sandwich on buttered toast with a glass of juice.

Picky Eaters

It is a fact of life that different children have different appetites and different attitudes toward food. Their taste buds and sensitivities to texture, temperature, and flavor are as diverse as the children themselves. That is just the way it is. So, if one can step back and be sensitive to a child's preferences, a lot of annoyance and confusion can be avoided.

Some of children's apparently ingrained preferences can be modified by early exposure to particular foods, but sometimes a little unintended coercion can turn distaste into a powerful food aversion. There is nothing more likely to make a child hate a food than having to eat it under less than ideal circumstances. For example, if a child were introduced to Jell-O when she was suffering from an intestinal flu, she might not want to see the stuff again for months, because she associates the nausea and vomiting from her illness with mounds of wobbly dessert. Parents have to be in tune to such idiosyncrasies and navigate around them. Remember too that there is virtually no food that a child *must* eat. If any food is presented as such, it becomes like medicine, and medicine is different from food. Also, cajoling a child to eat in exchange for favors becomes an escalating battle of wills, and *the child will win.* The little extra food consumed in exchange for the bribe is not worth the effort, and if the pattern is allowed to balloon, fruitless hours can be spent sitting in front of a plate when everyone could be doing something useful and constructive.

Experience has shown how resilient and flexible children are when it comes to maintaining a steady rate of growth and weight. Even picky eaters who limit themselves to four or five food items thrive just as healthily as their peers. It all evens out in the end. All a parent's incessant pressure produces is stronger resistance from the child: every meal becomes a battle and an unpleasant experience, repeated and reinforced day after day, the negative effects of which can be long lasting.

A Built-In "Calorie-Stat"

Because infants and children are programmed physiologically to consume their required calories, they will let you know when they are satisfied. The sensor for calories (or "calorie-stat," as in thermostat) probably gets signals through hormones transmitted both in the brain and in fat cells.

This is more complicated than it sounds, of course, but the bottom line is this: If you were to dilute a baby's formula, he would instinctively consume more ounces of it—just enough to make up for the calories that would have been lost in the watered-down version. The opposite is also true: try to enrich the formula with cereal, fat, or a supplement, and he will naturally decrease his intake to match his caloric need. It's a remarkable phenomenon, but it makes sense and can definitely help increase a parent's insight into feedings.

A child's weight usually at least doubles in the first six months of life and triples in the first year, gaining roughly a pound every two weeks in the first six months and then a pound a month until the first birthday. After age two, a child will gain only three to five pounds a year. Length increases by 50 percent

the first year, but does not double until age four; between age
two and puberty, children only grow about two inches *a year*.
Infants and young toddlers, then, need a very high-calorie diet
to sustain their rapid growth, and any child who continues that
level of consumption after age two risks gaining too much
weight.

APPROXIMATE DAILY CALORIC REQUIREMENTS BY AGE AND WEIGHT		
Age	Per Pound	Per Kilogram
Birth—1 year	50	110
1 to 3 years	45	100
4 to 6 years	40	90
7 to 10 years	30	70
11 to 14 years	20	50

Source: *Pediatric Nutrition Handbook*, 11th ed., 1998.

HELPFUL HINTS

- Be patient and keep your eyes on the bigger picture: Is she growing well? Is your doctor or caregiver happy about his progress? Are
  there any concerns about dehydration or iron deficiency? Is she
  fatigued or energetic?
- Remember that a child is allowed to have food preferences.
  Trying to impose yours might have the opposite of any intended
  effect.
- Make meals pleasant and enjoyable; don't bribe or threaten to
  remove privileges in an effort to make children eat.

- Avoid conflict, as it angers and depresses children: they are bound to react negatively.
- Serve manageable portions at meals, not impossibly large ones.
- Limit the amount of juice consumption: it might result in a dramatic new interest in eating.
- Don't promise dessert as a reward for cleaning the plate.

Nutrition in Adolescents

Accelerated weight gain and bone growth is to be expected during the adolescent years, which can start as early as age eleven, particularly in girls. The body is preparing for the reproductive tasks ahead, and it blossoms. The central control for this hormonal revolution is located both in the pituitary gland, which is found at the center of the brain, and in the peripheral glands—the adrenals and the male and female sex organs. These glands engage in a coordinated sequence aimed at increasing body fat and muscle. The results are always dramatic: if you don't see an adolescent for a week, you can tell they have grown since you saw them last!

Teenagers can have legendary appetites. Their insatiable hunger is aimed at taking in all the building blocks needed to build tissue, a process called the anabolic response. This is a time when overshooting caloric needs is the norm rather than the exception, and the sudden weight changes that can result are a reason why so many teenagers are upset about their bodies and wage a constant battle against the instinctive impulse to eat and eat.

Nutritionally, at least in this country, the teenager is at a clear disadvantage: because their schedules are tight and they never get enough sleep, they often skip breakfast and at lunch find their only choices to be among various fast foods, which offer excess saturated fats and too many calories. A family meal at dinnertime, when there is one, might not make up for all the shortcomings accrued during the day.

HELPFUL HINTS

- Teach by example: start encouraging good eating habits from the time children are very young.
- Make healthy choices at the supermarket.
- Avoid bringing home food you don't want children to eat.
- Cook balanced meals; don't rely on fast foods, if at all possible.
- Encourage physical activity, not necessarily competitive sports. Exercise together!
- Actively discourage uncontrolled television watching; set time rules early on.

EATING DISORDERS

As we are so painfully aware, adolescence is the time when eating disorders such as anorexia nervosa and bulimia can manifest themselves. Anorexia nervosa is a feeding disorder driven by deep psychological distortions in body image and self-worth, involving control issues and an unconscious attempt to prevent weight gain at all costs. It is a psychiatric disorder that can be devastating, and parents need to be on the lookout to recognize its early symptoms. Eating disorders affect girls much more frequently than boys, but male anorexia is not as rare as previously believed—up to 10 percent of boys may be affected, according to some reports. (For more information, see references in appendix.)

SIGNS OF ANOREXIA NERVOSA

- **An obsession with being fat**
- **An unrealistic image of oneself as actually being fat, when clearly this is not the case**
- **Emaciation (scrawniness)**
- **Exaggerated hyperactivity and involvement in physical activity aimed at burning energy**
- **Exaggerated interest in food preparation coupled with a marked restraint when it comes to eating**

The New Food Pyramid Explained

Providing nutritional advice to the population at large has been the task of the United States Department of Agriculture—a difficult job, since it means balancing ease of compliance by food producers with health-promoting principles. In the USDA's initial food pyramid, introduced in 1992, many compromises between these dual imperatives were made and the resulting simplifications provided scientifically unsound advice. Today, with current knowledge and with a better understanding of the factors contributing to improved cardiovascular health, revised recommendations are being offered.

The two major flaws in the old food pyramid were its assumptions that all fats were bad for you and all carbohydrates were good for you. Both were oversimplifications. In an attempt to promote decreased calorie consumption and lower Americans' risk of obesity, the original food pyramid recommended cutting back on fat intake. This should have produced the desired results: thinner people with less cardiovascular illness— lower incidence of heart disease, strokes, and hypertension. But as it turns out, not all fats are created equal, and some fats are actually very good for you. For example, monounsaturated fats, such as those in olive oil and polyunsaturated vegetable fats (in corn and safflower oils, for example), can improve the body's balance of "good cholesterol" (high-density lipoprotein, or HDL) to "bad cholesterol" (low-density lipoprotein, or LDL), and thus provide health benefits, even when the amounts con-

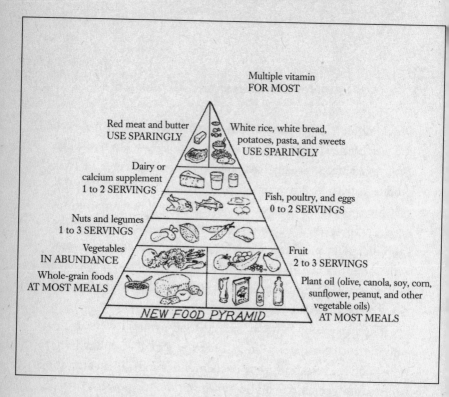

FIGURE #12 The New Food Pyramid

sumed exceed the initially recommended levels of 30 percent of the total daily calories. And population surveys and many clinical studies, in fact, do point to the beneficial effects of diets in which 40 percent of total daily calories come from certain "good" fats such as those in olive oil, many vegetable oils, and fish oils rich in omega-3 fatty acids (which are also found in walnuts).

In contrast, trans-unsaturated fatty acids (more simply referred to as trans-fatty acids) should be avoided. These "bad" fats are found in margarines and are commonly used in commercially baked and fried items. They are formed through a chemical process that converts liquid vegetable oils into solids, and they are particularly unhealthy because they not only increase the bad cholesterol in our bodies but also simultaneously decrease the good kind.

The concerns that the USDA's 1992 food pyramid raised over the last decade about the impact of dietary fat on obesity seem to have been unfounded, so new guidelines were issued in 2002. Today, the prevailing scientific wisdom holds that in order to prevent obesity, we should limit our *total* daily calories, not just the calories provided by fat. In fact, the new food pyramid recommends zero to two servings of fish, poultry, or eggs per day, as opposed to the two to three servings in the old pyramid, but liberalizes the consumption of plant oils like canola, soy, and sunflower at most meals. It also recommends one to three servings of nuts and legumes, as well as an abundance of vegetables, each day.

ORGANIC = HEALTHY?

As the popularity of organic food soars (it's a $9-billion-a-year industry), the differences between "organic" and "healthy" are becoming blurred. The companies promoting organic products are interested in creating the impression that organic always equals healthy, but this is not always the case.

Using the standards of the United States Department of Agriculture, the label "organic" only denotes that the product is as free as possible (95 percent, at least) from impurities such as hormones, antibiotics, pesticides, or genetic engineering. A healthy food, meanwhile, is one that confers health benefits, such as a decreased risk of heart disease or cancer.

Some organic cookies and snacks are promoted as being healthier than their nonorganic counterparts because they contain no trans-fatty acids and use pesticide-free ingredients. But don't forget that a calorie is a calorie, and that some of the supposedly healthy organic foods are just as fatty or sugary as any others. The fact that the ten teaspoons of sugar used to sweeten one can of soda are from organic sugarcane does not magically make the drink a recommended item for your child's (or your) diet.

Recommendations: read labels, understand the issues, choose wisely, and keep a balanced diet.

CARBOHYDRATES AND PROCESSED STARCHES

New research casts refined carbohydrates and processed starches in a negative light. As their metabolism can increase triglycerides (fat) in the blood, these types of carbohydrates are believed to be an important risk factor for cardiovascular disease. Furthermore, many studies have confirmed that the liberal intake of carbohydrates—which one would consume plentifully to satisfy the calorie requirements suggested by the old pyramid—is a major contributor to obesity and to the development of type-2 (late onset) diabetes in people who do not exercise and are overweight.

THE GLYCEMIC INDEX   Whole grains, legumes, and vegetables should be eaten liberally at most meals, while carbohydrate-rich, or starchy, items such as potatoes, white rice, white bread, and refined sugars are to be used in moderation. Excess consumption of these latter foods may promote obesity, as all have a high glycemic index.

Developed in 1981 by a team led by D. J. A. Jenkins, the glycemic index expresses the effects of a particular carbohydrate on blood glucose levels over a period of two hours, in comparison with the absorption of pure glucose (which has an index value of 100). How a carbohydrate is processed is one of the critical factors in determining its glycemic index. For example, white bread has a high glycemic index compared to whole wheat, oats, or bran. Similarly, white rice has a higher index than brown rice. High-glycemic food has been associated with an increased risk of diabetes, obesity, and cardiovascular disease.

Another important concept is the glycemic load, which measures the amount of a particular carbohydrate (with its specific glycemic index) consumed in a portion of food. Calculating the load has been shown to be useful in managing patients with diabetes and in weight-reduction programs. Among the foods with a high glycemic index are the refined starchy foods. Low-index foods include vegetables, most fruits, and legumes. Lower glycemic loads will help minimize quick swings in blood sugar, affecting insulin levels, which in turn increase hunger and can impact the body's processing of fat. People whose diets include high-glycemic foods are at greater risk for obesity than those who favor low-glycemic foods.

GLYCEMIC INDEXES AND GLYCEMIC LOADS FOR SELECTED FOODS

FOOD	GLYCEMIC INDEX	SERVING SIZE	GLYCEMIC LOAD
Instant rice	91	4 oz.	24.8
Baked potato	85	3.5 oz.	20.3
Corn flakes	84	7 oz.	21
Carrot	71	1.5 oz.	3.8
White bread	70	2 slices	21.0
Rye bread	65	2 slices	19.5
Muesli	56	3.5 oz.	16.8
Banana	53	5.5 oz.	13.3
Spaghetti	41	1.5 oz.	16.4
Apple	36	5.5 oz.	8.1
Lentils	29	3.5 oz.	5.7
Milk	27	7 oz.	3.2
Peanuts	14	1 oz.	0.7

Source: David S. Ludwig, "The Glycemic Index," *Journal of the American Medical Association* 283 (2002): 2,414.

FRUITS AND VEGETABLES

Fruits and vegetables continue to be recommended in the new pyramid, as they are an important source of folic acid, potassium, and vitamins. Folic acid protects against birth defects and against colon cancer, while potassium may also protect against cancer. Yet even if these benefits could not be solidly proven—and it is very difficult to carry out long-term studies that can pinpoint the beneficial, or detrimental, effects of a particular nutrient—eating fruits and vegetables should be encouraged, as they provide a natural source of essential vitamins.

Take note, however: a potato is a starch, despite its placement in the pyramid's vegetable group! Nuts, on the other hand, initially viewed with suspicion because of their high fat content, have recently been embraced because they are rich in polyunsaturated fats, omega-3 fatty acids, vitamins, and minerals—all well recognized for their protective properties. Not only that, but nuts satisfy the appetite and thus prevent us from eating excessive amounts of other foods that may not be as good for us.

MEATS AND PROTEIN

This brings us to protein. We need to make distinctions between protein sources. How different is red meat from fish, poultry, or even eggs? Very different, when you evaluate red meat's high saturated-fat and cholesterol contents. The new pyramid makes this distinction by separating recommendations for fish, poultry, and eggs (zero to two servings) from red meat and butter (use sparingly), whereas the old pyramid lumped them all together.

MILK AND DAIRY PRODUCTS

It is common knowledge that dairy products and milk are excellent sources of calcium, and it is a common belief that, as the advertisements say, "Milk is a Natural." The dairy industry has reinforced the belief that milk is an excellent food and that its consumption should be encouraged. And certainly, dairy products are a generous source of protein and also an easily available source of calcium and vitamin D. (A word of caution: Allergy to cow's milk protein and intolerance to milk sugar [lactose] are both common problems in our society.) What do we recommend for children? After age three, only skim milk should be offered; there is no need for all the saturated fat in whole milk or even 1 percent milk. Excessive milk consumption needs to be avoided—not more than sixteen to twenty ounces a day—because milk satisfies the appetite and decreases interest in other iron-rich foods such as cereals and meats, putting the child at risk for developing iron-deficiency anemia.

The whole point of breaking down the old food pyramid and rebuilding it was to highlight and correct the many health beliefs and habits that needed revising. While the USDA's 1992 food pyramid had blocks that promoted good health, those benefits were too often counterbalanced by others that perpetuated old disproven ideas. Although the effort was well intentioned, the goal to improve the general health of the population (not specifically children) went unrealized.

Yet while the new pyramid offers significant improvement, it is important to remember that newer studies suggest that lifestyle changes and not only diet are fundamental to good health. Successful ingredients include increased exercise, not smoking, adherence to a balanced diet rich in wholesome foods, fruits, vegetables, and healthy fats, and avoidance of obesity by a decrease in total calories consumed. This is a continuing field of study, one that is valuable to keep an eye on, but using your own common sense—based on the latest data available—goes a long way!

11

Why Does the Tummy Hurt? Pinpointing Pain

CHAPTER 3

Why Does the Intestine Hurt?

Location, Duration, and Quality of Pain

The main goal of this book is to make sense of children's common complaints of abdominal pain, and, as we said in chapter 1, knowledge empowers. And nowhere is such empowerment more welcome than when it helps a parent's self-confidence when shouldering responsibility for the well-being of his or her child.

This chapter will describe the reasons why children develop stomachaches and the importance of paying attention to the location, duration, and quality, or character, of the pain. Because pain does not come out of the blue and is linked to other important and telling symptoms, we will also try to encourage you to look beyond the pain and see the larger picture: the context in which pain occurs. The following are a few questions you should ask yourself when faced with the complaint of "my tummy hurts":

▌ Did the pain last a short time?
▌ Did the pain come and go?
▌ Did the pain interfere with the child's activities?
▌ Was the pain accompanied by nausea or vomiting?
▌ If there was vomiting, what was brought up?

▌ Did the pain improve with time? Spiral up?

▌ Was the pain accompanied by a fever?

The answers to these questions will help you focus on the details that help us in our task as medical detectives. You also need to be a good detective, and in many ways you have the advantage: you see your child every day and night, you can observe his reactions to food or to activities, and you can sense whether stress or other sources of tension or emotional upset may be involved. With a cool head, you will be able to take the first steps toward understanding what could be triggering your child's moaning or groaning.

Why Does the Intestine Hurt?

In simple terms, there are four main mechanisms for intestinal pain:

☹ Overstretching (distension) of the walls of the bowel

☹ Decreased blood flow (ischemia) to the bowel

☹ Irritation caused by acid in the stomach or esophagus

☹ Supersensitive gut (visceral hypersensitivity), a state of intense responsiveness to what most people consider a normal sensation in the bowel

OVERSTRETCHING (DISTENSION)

The overstretching of the wall of the intestine is picked up by pain sensors sandwiched between the intestine's muscle layers.

They are very sensitive, and for a good reason: the stretching of the intestine can be the early warning of obstruction, a potentially serious condition that needs to be addressed without delay.

It is no wonder that systems aimed at alerting us that stretching is taking place should be highly developed. In evolutionary terms, such sensors are an early-warning system for life-threatening situations, and they hence play a major role in survival. Every one of our hollow organs, including the gallbladder and bile ducts, the kidney and its draining ureters, the uterus, and the pancreatic ducts, shares this important property.

DECREASED BLOOD FLOW (ISCHEMIA)

Decreased blood flow to the bowel (ischemia) is the equivalent of an intestinal heart attack—think of it as a "gut attack"—except that reasons for the lessened blood and oxygen supply are totally different in children than they are in adults. In adults, heart-muscle and intestinal ischemia is caused by arteriosclerosis, or what is commonly known as "hardening of the arteries."

By contrast, ischemia in children is most commonly related to congenital problems that allow the blood supply to the intestine to be "pinched off" (for example by a volvulus: literally, a twisting of the intestine around itself) or acquired conditions in which the intestine can telescope on itself, trapping the veins and arteries (intussusception).

Both overstretching and poor blood supply are potentially serious conditions that might even require surgery to correct. Therefore, our initial questions about children's stomachaches are always aimed at ruling out this possibility.

IRRITATION: DAMAGE TO THE INTESTINE'S PROTECTIVE COATING

Normally, the lining of the digestive tract is covered by a protective coating of mucus. This mucus is manufactured by the cells lining the bowel, all the way from the mouth to the anus, and its job is to keep bacteria and parasites away, lubricate the tract, and provide a buffer between the bowel wall and the highly acidic gastric juices that might injure it. (If the levels of acidity in the stomach are strong enough to corrode metal, what would prevent them from eating right through the intestinal wall? In a word, mucus.) It is a dynamic layer, always changing and being replenished when food, bacteria, or other irritants disrupt it.

Sometimes this protection fails, and a disruption of the coating layer follows, causing irritation. If the damage is not repaired fast enough, an ulcer will develop, exposing nerve endings to the irritating effects of acid and other chemicals. As those nerves are inflamed, we experience pain. The bowel can also be irritated by chemicals released in the intestinal cells themselves as a result of immune-system damage, as seen in cases of food allergy, or when parasites invade the lining and travel through or settle in the intestine.

SUPERSENSITIVE GUT (VISCERAL HYPERSENSITIVITY)

A person with a supersensitive gut feels acutely what most people would consider a normal sensation in the bowel. The condition can develop after certain infections, or for no apparent reason. It is an important factor at play in children with certain chronic abdominal pain. (See chapter 4 for a detailed description of visceral hypersensitivity and the role it plays in functional pain).

Describing Pain

What can you tell your pediatrician or health care provider to help sort out the possible causes for the pain? How can you help provide clues about the level of urgency of your child's complaint?

How to help? Review the following and provide information on them as accurately as possible:

- Onset of pain (when it started) and changes with time
- Location and referral pattern of the pain
- Quality and changing character of the pain

Let's address each one in turn.

ONSET OF PAIN

This is a key question in the evaluation of any pain, as it ascertains the time at which the problem began to appear. In the case of bellyaches, it helps clarify whether the child was perfectly well before she started crying, and it can also establish whether the complaint had been going on for a while but wasn't previously serious enough to prompt a visit to a doctor. For example, asking when the pain started and getting a response like, "Oh, I don't know exactly, probably a few months ago . . . I'm not sure" is very different from "She was playing with her friends after lunch, and at 2:00 P.M. she came running to me grabbing her tummy."

Being able to provide an accurate chronology of the complaints is as important as pinpointing the onset of the pain. We need to be as focused as possible, and an exact history of the issue can help narrow the range of problems and help us reach the right diagnosis quickly. In this regard, you must learn, or recall, what happened before and after you heard the complaint or noticed there was something bothering her: Was it after a meal? What did she eat? Was there anything unusual about the diet, compared to her routine? Was he hungry? Did he feel like going to the bathroom? Was the bowel movement different? At the time, was there anyone sick at home? Does anyone at home have similar symptoms? What happened next?

As you try to present the sequence of events, you start to build a chain of possible causes and effects. Questions like those previously suggested lead to more specific probing and focus: Was it the milk he had at dinner? Was it the passage of a very hard bowel movement? Was it the antibiotics he was receiving for the sore throat? Did he drink apple cider during the school trip? Perhaps too much fruit salad for dessert?

The Symptom Diary

Questions to Ask: Onset of Pain
- When did the pain start?
- Did the pain start suddenly or did it build up over time? If the latter, how long has it been an issue?
- Did anything specific and unusual precede or follow the pain? Was there a diet change? Did the child experience a difficult bowel movement?
- What other symptoms accompanied the onset of pain? Was there nausea? Vomiting? Fever?
- Have there been any similar episodes in the past? When? How were they resolved? What was done?
- Is there anyone with similar complaints in the household? Any history of travel? Of trauma?
- How did the pain evolve? Did it improve over time? Worsen?
- What happened between onset and change?

LOCATION OF PAIN

Pain in the general area of the tummy—a very vague and poorly defined geographic area for any child—can originate in any of the following areas:

- The intestinal tract and its associated organs (liver, gallbladder, pancreas, spleen)
- The peritoneum (the fine membrane that covers all the organs and the lining of the abdominal cavity itself)
- Nonintestinal organs, e.g., kidneys, ureters, bladder, and spine

Interestingly, pain from the lungs (when inflamed by pneumonia or in spasm during severe asthma), or even the heart, can be felt in the abdomen. This phenomenon of feeling pain away from the original organ responsible for the pain is called referred pain.

The Symptom Diary

Questions to Ask: Location of the Pain
- Where exactly does it hurt? Point with your finger (or hand, as the case may be)
- Does it hurt more (or less) when you move? Lay down? Cough? Urinate? Have a bowel movement?
- Does the pain move around? Where does it refer to? (See "Referred Pain" below.)
- Has the location changed since symptoms started? How? When?
- Does anything else hurt?

REFERRED PAIN   Referred pain is easily understood when one recalls that during the fetal development the nerves appear in segments and travel some distance, sometimes rotating in the process, so that at the end, the initial place from which the nerves originated is not necessarily close to the organ for which it will send signals to the brain.

This same principle explains the pattern and location of pain from an inflamed appendix. No matter where the appendix is in the body, the initial pain of appendicitis will be felt around the belly button. Later, the location of the pain will depend on where the actual appendix irritates the lining of the abdomen; it can be in the right lower quadrant but also may be experienced in the back, right upper quadrant, or even next to the rectum. (See figure 13.) The following table will help you identify the most common "referred pain" areas for many medical and surgical problems. (It is important to note, though, that in general, the more diffuse pain is—the more it is spread out all over and not pinpointed—or the closer it is centered around the belly button, the less likely it is one of the conditions possibly requiring surgery. But clearly, this is a determination that only your doctor is qualified to make!)

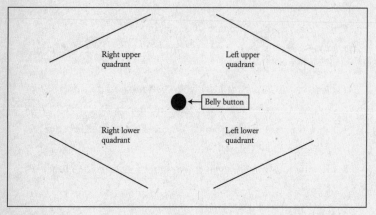

FIGURE #13 The Four Quadrants of the Abdomen

This simple diagram helps understand the locations of pain listed in the Table on page 53. The upper angles illustrate the rib margins, while the lower angles delineate the hips.

PAIN LOCATION QUADRANTS AND POSSIBLE CAUSES

LOCATION QUADRANTS	POSSIBLE CAUSES OF PAIN
Right upper	Cholecystitis (gallbladder inflammation); gallstones; gastritis; peptic ulcer disease; pelvic inflammatory disease; pneumonia; peritonitis
Left upper	Gastritis; peptic ulcer disease; esophagitis; pneumonia; spleen hemorrhage or injury
Middle upper	Gastritis; gastroesophageal reflux or esophagitis; esophageal narrowing or swallowed foreign body; pancreatitis; peptic ulcer disease
Right mid- or lower	Appendicitis; inflammatory bowel disease; kidney stones; kidney infection; obstruction of the ureter; ovarian torsion, cyst, or abscess; pelvic inflammatory disease
Left mid- or lower	Kidney stones; kidney obstruction; pyelonephritis (inflammation or infection of the kidneys); ovarian torsion
Around belly button	Constipation; functional abdominal pain; intestinal flu; intussusception (telescoping of the intestine); inflammatory bowel disease; irritable bowel syndrome; lactose intolerance
Below the belly button	Bladder infection or obstruction; constipation; inflammatory bowel disease; irritable bowel syndrome; pelvic inflammation

When the source of pain is actually in the digestive tract itself, it is by nature deep, diffuse, and difficult to pinpoint. Pain receptors in the peritoneum, muscles, joints, and skin are easily located, but a tummy ache, on the other hand, is more spread out, because of the overlapping network of nerves in the intestine and its organs. Describing pain is thus sometimes quite difficult, even for a grownup. Imagine asking a young child to do so, or, worse yet, expecting a parent to describe what they think their infant or child's complaints really feel like!

In general, however, we can gather important information by trying to determine whether pain is intermittent or steady. Intermittent, or colicky, pain, implies muscle contraction in a hollow organ. This applies to pain from the intestine, as well as pain from the ureters or bile ducts, as when passing a kidney stone or a gallstone. The stretch receptors are distended by a pocket of gas in the intestine that causes the muscles to cramp, or by inflammation deep in the intestine releasing irritants that result in spasms. Colicky pain can be quite intense. If this is accompanied by nausea and vomiting, we need to consider the possibility of an obstruction, although nausea can be associated with strong pain from any number of sources. Colicky pain experienced while "funny gurgling noises" are heard from inside suggests that the cramps are caused by poorly absorbed food and fluid swishing and swashing with each muscle contraction.

Steady pains are often caused by irritation of parts of the intestine or by distension or inflammation of one of the solid organs, such as the liver, spleen, or pancreas. The pain of pancreatitis, for example, is an intense, sometimes debilitating and excruciating, steady sensation felt in the pit of the stomach and typically going toward the back—"like a knife was being plunged right through me," as one teenaged patient so vividly described.

These are just brief descriptions of conditions causing very different types of pain. The message is that by listening carefully to these descriptions we can begin to think of what could be causing the pain, and with more pointed questions, we can come closer to a possible diagnosis. Reaching the right diagnosis is crucial before proper care can be instituted. Evaluating all of the information gathered during the history and complementing it with selected laboratory and imaging studies helps the specialist understand the nature of the problem.

Therefore, medical history, physical examination, and a selected choice of laboratory and diagnostic tests are the three pillars upon which a more certain diagnosis stands, but only positive response to treatment confirms the diagnosis.

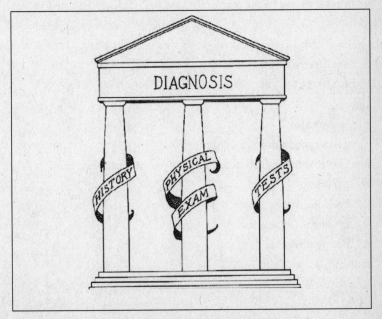

FIGURE #14   Three Pillars of Diagnosis

Evaluating Pain

When you call your pediatrician or health care provider to report the onset of pain in your child, one of the first judgments they will make is whether the situation is urgent, requiring a referral to the emergency room, or one that can wait for a scheduled appointment. It may help to keep in mind some of the conditions that commonly cause pain in various age groups but *do not* require surgical treatment.

IN INFANTS

- Colic/fussiness
- Formula intolerance (carbohydrate malabsorptions, protein allergy)
- Gastroenteritis (intestinal infections caused by viruses or bacteria)
- Rectal fissure (small tear in the skin and folds of the anus)

IN TODDLERS, PREADOLESCENTS, AND ADOLESCENTS

- Indigestion
- Constipation or fecal impaction
- Gastroenteritis (infection caused by viruses, bacteria, or parasites)
- Food poisoning
- Hepatitis
- Pancreatitis

RED FLAGS: Contact Your Doctor Without Delay When . . .

There are times when a stomachache is accompanied by certain features that we consider red flags. When red flags occur, we know that serious reasons may underlie the problem, and you need to act promptly.

RED FLAGS

- Vomiting of bile (green or yellowish-green stomach contents)
- Vomiting bright-red blood
- Vomiting coffee ground–like material (the "coffee grounds" are actually digested blood)
- Unexplained lethargy or sleepiness alternating with bouts of crampy abdominal pains, with or without vomiting
- Nighttime pain that wakes your child from a deep sleep
- Acute pain with abdominal bloating or distension
- Painful swelling in the groin or belly button that cannot be gently squeezed back
- Pain aggravated by any movement or makes the tummy feel hard as a board
- Pain accompanied by high fevers
- Pain accompanied by severe loss of appetite, inability to drink sufficiently, and dehydration (indicated by sunken eyes, dry mouth, no tears, sleepiness, and weakness)
- Pain associated with urination
- Pain associated with passage of dark (sticky black) stools
- Passage of bloody or maroon-colored stools, even if not associated with pain
- Pain and unusual pallor

- Pain and altered mental status (lethargy, delirium, disorientation, uncharacteristic aggression, for example)

All of these symptoms reflect the presence of either an obstruction (which can cause the vomiting of bile) or damage to the intestinal lining resulting in bleeding, ischemia, or peritonitis. The presence of mental changes—disorientation, aggressiveness, hallucination—can point to blood poisoning from a damaged intestine or from obstruction, perforation, or dehydration.

As you can see, these are all potentially alarming conditions, but they are manageable if help is sought immediately. Don't be shy about reporting your concerns; don't feel bad about disturbing the doctor or worrying what he or she will think of you for feeling alarmed. It is easier to confirm that there's nothing to worry about than to be confronted with a far more advanced and complicated condition that could have been avoided. Still, sometimes surgery is unavoidable. The most common conditions that might require surgery include the following.

APPENDICITIS   Inflammation of the appendix, the wormlike extension at the beginning of the large intestine. It is the most common reason for emergency surgery in children.

GALLSTONES   OR   GALLBLADDER   INFLAMMATION Gallstones formed from superconcentrated bile. Inflammation of the gallbladder by bacteria or impaired blood flow disrupts the normal flow of bile.

INCARCERATED HERNIA   A loop of intestine, intestinal fat, or even an ovary can find its way through a weak spot in the muscles of the abdominal wall. The most common hernias are those found in the groin (inguinal) or the belly button (umbilical). If the loop cannot return back to its place, it becomes "incarcerated," resulting in swelling and impaired blood flow.

INTUSSUSCEPTION   The telescoping of one segment of intestine into another next to it. This causes a blockage, and if it lasts long, it can damage the wall and perforate. It is the most common cause of intestinal obstruction in the first year of life.

MALROTATION OR VOLVULUS   The twisting of the intestine around its main blood supply caused by a failure of the intestine to be properly anchored during its development.

MECKEL'S DIVERTICULUM   A small pouch usually found about a foot away from the end of the small intestine. It can become inflamed; up to half of these inflammations are caused by the acid that it produces itself. If the pouch collapses into the intestine, blockage may result. It is the most common birth defect of the intestine.

OBSTRUCTING KIDNEY STONE   A stone moving from the kidney to be expelled from the body can become stuck along the way, in the ureter as it exits the kidney or as it enters the bladder. Pain is intense, radiates down the groin, and is felt on the flank and back. Nausea is also common.

PEPTIC ULCER   An ulcer caused by stomach acid irritating the stomach lining to the point where it creates a small crater. In addition to pain, this can result in bleeding and in obstruction of the stomach outlet. Many ulcers are caused by infection with *H. pylori*, a corkscrew-shaped bacterium that can inflame the stomach lining (see chapter 17), or by aspirin-like irritant medications.

In subsequent chapters, we will describe some of the important pediatric conditions that cause tummy aches, how to recognize them, and how to respond. Just as you had to learn certain facts about your car and certain rules about driving, you have to know certain things about your child and his body. Here, too, information about your child's "engine," its various parts and potential problem areas, is needed to plan proper care.

CHAPTER 4

Chronic Pain and How Emotions
Affect the Gut

The study of how the enteric nervous system (ENS), the "brain in the gut," responds to painful triggers and how pain is processed before we actually experience it is a growing area of research. Over the last decade, we have witnessed a revolution in our understanding of the intricate mechanisms involved and have been able to shed light on the interplay between the immune system, pain receptors in the gut, and parts of the brain that integrate and process painful sensations. As a result of all this work, we can now begin to explain why the intestine can continue to hurt even after the original reason for the pain has cleared and why some people appear to be especially sensitive when it comes to intestinal discomfort. In this chapter, I will review the wide range of clinical presentations of children with chronic abdominal pain and the newest classification of these conditions. Visceral hypersensitivity and functional pain, two important concepts central to our ability to diagnose and treat children with chronic abdominal pain, will be discussed, as will the three main functional disorders in children: irritable bowel syndrome, functional dyspepsia, and functional abdominal pain syndrome.

How We Experience Pain

Every person experiences pain differently, because the body can reprocess pain signals in many ways. For example, the pain signal may be influenced by a person's emotional state: when someone is injured but is also frightened or excited, he may not be aware of the injury right away. You've probably experienced this yourself. You'll notice a bruise one day and have no memory of how it happened. The reverse is also true. If a child is totally focused on an injection he is about to receive, he will react to it more intensely. Thus, pain is always subjective and cannot be quantified. A parent may say, "Come on, that didn't hurt," but, although needles used in injections are tiny, some children react to them and others don't. For children who are needlephobic, the fear and anxiety brought on by the prospect of an injection are very real and intensify any pain they may feel.

Pain in the intestine is very different from pain in a joint or pain from the stab of a needle. In the intestine, "stretch receptors" generate painful sensations when activated by gas distension or muscle cramping, and the nerve messages that register this pain in the brain go on quite a different journey from those induced by a needle prick. As the sensation from the gut is processed on the way to the brain, there are many opportunities for the initial signal to be modified. Depending on the path it takes, it can either be weakened or intensified, and the level of pain it produces will be perceived accordingly.

This is an important new understanding: that pain is fine-tuned on its way to the brain was not known until recently. This signal modification is part of the communication that goes on within the nervous system as a whole. There is communication between the high centers in the brain and the gut as well as among the millions of cells in the ENS up and down the gut.

Signals also pass between the gut and the spine and from the spine up to the higher centers. This amounts to a lot of chattering, and it makes intestinal pain a difficult target. Furthermore, we now know that the constant firing of painful sensations can actually make some nerve cells sprout additional nerve routes, leaving the switch for pain on even when the original injury has cleared!

Visceral Hypersensitivity

One of the main causes of chronic intestinal pain is visceral hypersensitivity. This intimidating phrase needs some explanation: *viscera* generally includes the gastrointestinal organs we described in chapter 1, while *hypersensitivity* connotes an exaggerated pain response to a particular stimulus. In basic terms, then, the condition may be called supersensitive gut.

When we are healthy, our tolerance for pain is high enough that we are not at all aware of our gut's functioning. Sometimes at night we might hear gurgles or notice something moving around, but this doesn't hit the brain with the urgency of a warning signal. The intestine is constantly stretching and filling with gas and fluid. Most of the time we don't feel this regular peristalsis, but in people who are primed and hypersensitive, it will be perceived as pain.

A supersensitive gut is a characteristic of many functional intestinal pains. In one research study, for example, adult subjects with irritable bowel syndrome (IBS) had a balloon placed in the small intestine, esophagus, or stomach. As the balloon was inflated, the subject was asked to indicate when they first felt pain and how strong it was. In the subjects with IBS, the upper limit of pain was substantially lower than in people who didn't have IBS. Consequently, because of this hypersensitivity, people with IBS are more likely to experience normal distension of the intestine as pain.

Functional Pain

Functional abdominal pain—bellyaches that seem to occur for no apparent reason—is common, and most children who go to the doctor with chronic abdominal pain actually have a functional disorder, meaning that while they don't have a disease, their system is not functioning well. There is no underlying blockage, inflammation, or other physical explanation for the complaint; the pain stems from a disruption in the key pain sensors or the hypersensitivity phenomenon previously described. And although there is nothing detectable, that does *not* imply that there is nothing wrong. There is, and it is hidden deep in the subtle workings of the interconnected cells of the brain and enteric nervous system. The pain is not imagined: it is real.

So, when a parent sees her child miserable, crying, bent over in pain, and nauseated, then clearly there *is* something wrong even if it is not readily apparent. In such cases, it is crucial that the physician relay unequivocally to parents that there is a problem in the way things are working. Parents should pass this acknowledgment and recognition on to the child.

RECURRENT ABDOMINAL PAIN

In 1958, two British pediatricians, John Apley and Nora Naish, described the phenomenon of recurrent abdominal pain of childhood. Apley was the first to establish criteria to define it as a distinct syndrome: at least three bouts of pain in the abdomen over three months in the last year, with each episode severe enough to affect the child's daily activities. Research since has found that RAP, as it is known, affects perhaps 10 to 20 percent of school-age children.

Apley's work was groundbreaking, in that it anticipated more recent descriptions of functional pain. Among his most significant conclusions was a "negative evidence of any physical association with the pains, and the positive evidence of frequent emotional disturbances" in patients with RAP.

Years later, at the 1988 International Congress of Gastroenterologists, held in Rome, Italy, a set of diagnostic criteria for irritable bowel syndrome was presented. The project was expanded to encompass all functional gastrointestinal disorders and the work, now known collectively as Rome I, was published in 1992. An updated set of criteria, Rome II, was published in 2000. The diagnostic criteria are now stricter than those proposed by Apley, and coordinating committees established in 2001 for Rome III continue the work. Among other refinements, the new criteria distinguish among a number of types of functional abdominal pain. Also included, for the first time, are symptomologies of the functional disorders affecting children.

As delineated by Rome II, there are three major functional pain syndromes, all of which can affect children: irritable bowel syndrome (IBS), functional dyspepsia, and functional abdominal pain syndrome.

IRRITABLE BOWEL SYNDROME

Probably the most common functional pain syndrome, IBS has been diagnosed in children as young as seven or eight years of age. Studies indicate that anywhere from 6 to 14 percent of adolescents exhibit symptoms consistent with IBS.

SYMPTOMS   According to the Rome II criteria, irritable bowel syndrome is defined by the following:

- At least three months of abdominal pain in the previous year (months can be nonconsecutive)
- Pain relieved by having a bowel movement
- Pain that occurs together with a change in the appearance of the stool or in the form or frequency of the stool
- No underlying identifiable structural or medical problems

Irritable bowel syndrome is associated with going to the bathroom. Children will complain of stooling difficulties, and of having diffuse pain that is clearly not related to a parasite or to inflammatory bowel disease. Often they also report the sensation of not having moved their bowels enough, or that their stools are hard and pelletlike when they finally pass them. Also, diarrhea might alternate with constipation. Some patients with IBS will break into sweats, look pale, and feel nauseated when experiencing the pain, and they often will lie down and hold themselves, moaning and groaning. Sometimes, parents are worried when there is mucus in the stool. They shouldn't be. Mucus is a natural lubricant of the bowel, and it is secreted when stools become hard and difficult to pass.

Irritable bowel symptoms can have a serious impact on a child's quality of life. Children, specifically adolescents, may become reluctant to go anywhere for fear of not having easy access to a bathroom. Fearing that they might get an episode of cramps in the middle of an activity or a bus ride, they begin to avoid school activities or outings. They can also become self-conscious and insecure in their daily activities.

DIAGNOSIS   The key to making a positive diagnosis of IBS is identifying the typical pattern of symptoms. At the same time, we look for clues that might point to an underlying problem masquerading as chronic pain with intermittent diarrhea and constipation. It is always reassuring in these instances to see that despite weeks, or months, of not feeling well, the child is growing well and has no other complaints. This is a strong indication that no other problem is present. Laboratory tests are also used to confirm that no chronic condition exists. Still, parents and doctors must be vigilant. Three red flags to watch out for are:

- Delay in puberty or delay in growth accompanying the chronic pain
- Signs, such as fevers, blood in the stools, or vomiting of blood, that the pain is causing inflammation
- Disrupted sleep: the child wakes up in the middle of the night from the pain

In the clinical workup of any child with chronic pain, we will always include a detailed dietary history, because quite often it will offer clues to a possible source of the complaints. Lactose intolerance, for example, is always a possibility, as is excessive fiber consumption. If indicated, a change in diet or further specific tests will be recommended. Also, if the pain exhibits features of stomach irritation or reflux disease, an endoscopy (described in chapter 5) might be scheduled after an appropriate medication trial. If blood accompanies the abnormal bowel movements, or if other features in the history suggest an organic problem, a colonoscopy may also be scheduled. An important guideline is that the workup is individualized: no two patients are exactly the same, and no standard set of tests is indicated for everyone.

TREATMENT It is important for you, as the parent, to understand that the pain caused by irritable bowel syndrome is real—it's not in the child's head; it's not psychosomatic or otherwise imagined. It's as real as any bad headache. Yet although we know it's real, we don't have good medications to offer for its treatment. However, once the diagnosis of IBS is made, we work closely with the parents or caregivers to manage the pain effectively.

The time-honored treatment of irritable bowel includes an increase in dietary fiber. This is particularly useful for those patients who have hard, pelletlike stools. A lack of natural bulk is believed to contribute to the dysfunction in IBS, and increasing the volume of the stool tends to make the colon's contractions less spastic. Although the introduction of supplementary fiber into the diet should be done very slowly and carefully, do not overdo it. Excessive fiber will result in worse bellyaches, from sudden exposure to larger amounts of these complex sugars and accompanying changes in the bacteria of the intestine. Increasing the fiber intake slowly to allow bacteria to adjust to the new load of complex sugar will avoid this pitfall.

An easy formula for calculating the recommended amount of fiber supplement for a child is the age in years plus five grams (remember, thirty grams equal one ounce). A twelve-year-old then, should receive seventeen grams, or approximately half an ounce, of fiber daily. Over-the-counter fiber supplements containing psyllium (fleawort seed) are easy for the parent to give, but not always as easy for the child to swallow. Sold in powdered form, these products must be stirred in liquid and drunk right away. Otherwise they absorb the liquid, swell, and become, as children put it, "gross."

In addition to psyllium, soluble fiber is now available in juice and powder form in such products as Juice Plus Fiber and Benefiber, making it much easier to take than bran flakes added to hamburgers or other foods. Older children, and especially teenagers, prefer to take their fiber supplements in pill form (as Fibercon or the new Metamucil tablets, for example).

If the pain continues to disturb normal function even after the introduction of fiber, a specialist might recommend a trial of a tricyclic antidepressant such as amitriptyline. Such medication addresses the source of the problem: the abnormal perception of pain. (Although the common perception is that antidepressants are only for the treatment of emotional and mental issues, parents and patients need to understand that nerve endings in the gut and the transmission and perception by the brain are the target of these particular medications.)

IRRITABLE BOWEL SYNDROME: ONLY THE GUT HURTS

Patients who suffer from irritable bowel syndrome are not hypersensitive to *all* stimuli. They are not "wimps." Studies on their perception of pain when their hands are immersed in ice water, for example, show that subjects with IBS have a *higher* threshold for ice-water immersion compared to the population as a whole. They are in some ways tougher, less sensitive to pain that does not emanate from their bowels. What they have is a very specific gut hypersensitivity.

FUNCTIONAL DYSPEPSIA

Dyspepsia is recurrent pain in the upper abdomen, just under the ribs, in the area we commonly know as the pit of the stomach. It is a functional pain because, although it might feel much the same, it is not caused by hyperacidity or a bacterial infection. This pain is localized in the same place as pain caused by inflammation of the stomach or reflux disease, with all the features one sees when the esophagus or stomach are irritated, but, by definition, there is in this case no evidence of ulcers or any other physical cause for the persistent symptoms.

SYMPTOMS   In children mature enough to provide an accurate pain history, we look for the following symptoms to diagnose functional dyspepsia:

- At least twelve weeks (not necessarily consecutive) of discomfort
- Persistent or recurrent pain or discomfort centered in the upper abdomen (above the belly button)
- No evidence of physical disease that is likely to explain the symptoms, as determined by tests that could include an upper endoscopy
- No evidence that dyspepsia is relieved by defecation or is associated with the onset of a change in stool frequency or stool form (in other words, no evidence that the problem is irritable bowel syndrome)

DIAGNOSIS   When a patient's symptomatology matches that of functional dyspepsia, the next step is to diagnose which of two major types of functional dyspepsia is present: ulcer-like dyspepsia or dysmotility-like dyspepsia.

In cases of ulcer-like dyspepsia, the pain feels like an ulcer or reflux. Sometimes the pain is temporarily relieved with food or acid suppression, but when we investigate further and look for any evidence of acid irritation (by endoscopy, for example), no inflammation is found. This condition might be caused by muscle tension and irritated nerve endings or perhaps by abnormal production of chemicals in the nerves. We just don't know the reasons yet.

Dysmotility-like dyspepsia is characterized by nausea and bloating and a sense of being full after just a few bites of food. There might also be retching and vomiting. These complaints are quite different from the more localized pain in the pit of the stomach seen in ulcer-like dyspepsia.

TREATMENT   One of the initial steps in the treatment of functional dyspepsia is to use medications that suppress acidity, although they might not always provide full relief. At the same, it is important to modify the diet by decreasing the intake of fatty, fried foods that may be hard to digest. It is well known that stomach emptying is slowed down by fatty foods, so it is not surprising that this sort of diet modification might provide some relief. Also, avoiding medicines like aspirin and ibuprofen, which irritate the stomach, might help some patients with ulcer-like dyspepsia.

In addition, we now know that certain antidepressants may prove useful for this kind of functional upper-gastrointestinal disorder. At dosages lower than would be prescribed for depression, they can change the way the nervous system in the bowel works and may even affect the way the brain receives sensations of pain coming from the enteric nervous system.

FUNCTIONAL ABDOMINAL PAIN SYNDROME

The third manifestation of recurrent abdominal pain is functional abdominal pain syndrome, in which a school-age child or adolescent will have continuous pain that nothing seems to help. The child will say her pain rates a ten on a ten-point scale, all day long. Even if it might seem like an exaggeration, it is important to realize that the child is not malingering, complaining in pursuit of a secondary gain, or trying to avoid responsibilities: she is honestly feeling what she perceives to be a terrible pain, and we have to believe that she is feeling it all the time.

SYMPTOMS   We think that functional abdominal pain syndrome is another manifestation of disruption in both the enteric nervous system and the communication between the gut and brain, all complicated, and perhaps perpetuated, by the stresses of feeling sick. This pain is slightly different from that caused by irritable bowel syndrome or dyspepsia in that it doesn't have an association with stooling and isn't located in the upper stomach. The pain is more diffuse, centering on the belly button and spreading across the abdomen. In addition to abdominal pain, other complaints, such as dizziness, headaches, or leg pains, are often present and serious incapacitation is not unusual in cases of functional abdominal pain syndrome.

DIAGNOSIS   According to the Rome II criteria, functional abdominal pain syndrome is diagnosed when all of the following symptoms are present for at least six months:

- Continuous or nearly continuous abdominal pain
- No or only occasional relationship of pain with physiological events such as eating, defecation, or menses
- Some loss of daily functioning
- The pain is not faked

- Insufficient criteria for other functional gastrointestinal disorders that would explain the abdominal pain

TREATMENT   Since fully 95 percent of the serotonin in the body is manufactured in the gut, antidepressants based on serotonin reuptake are somehow effective there, working to modify pain perception. Some of the selective serotonin reuptake inhibitors (SSRIs), such as Prozac and Paxil, are also frequently used. Other medications in the class of anticonvulsants, among them gabapentin (Neurontin) or carbamazepine (Tegretol), and even antihypertensive drugs, such as clonidine (Catapres), can be useful in some patients.

To improve the overall condition of children with this debilitating form of chronic abdominal pain, we recommend these three steps:

- Modify activities as much as possible to allow the child to continue functioning.
- Return the child to a regular schedule as soon as possible.
- Involve behavioral medical specialists. They can teach self-hypnosis, biofeedback, breathing techniques, imaging—any number of techniques that can help to modify pain and foster a return to more normal function.

The following two relatively more rare conditions of functional pain, aerophagia and abdominal migraine, complete the classification of functional abdominal pain in children proposed by the Rome II panel of experts.

AEROPHAGIA (AIR SWALLOWING)

Aerophagia is the name given to a tendency of children (or adults) to swallow air in excessive amounts. Those with the condition are constantly belching and their bellies can become alarmingly swollen (distended) as the day goes on. During sleep they deflate, so feeling better by morning.

Jason made an excellent first impression when he walked into the office with his concerned parents. A tall and muscular teenager, he projected mischief with a twinkle in his eyes and did not seem particularly worried about coming for a medical consultation—I was his "third opinion," and he was enjoying the attention even while he did want to solve the problem. As his parents described Jason's "gas problem," he provided a vivid soundtrack: loud, explosive belches resounded every few minutes. "That's what they mean," his face said. His parents' faces were a mix of embarrassment and despair.

The treatment focused on teaching Jason to recognize that he was gulping air without fully realizing it and recommending specific breathing exercises to control this tendency. The good news is that Jason did try the breathing exercises, and they helped eradicate his socially inappropriate habits . . . to his own and his parents' relief.

ABDOMINAL MIGRAINE

Abdominal migraine is a rare condition characterized by episodes of severe abdominal pain that are sometimes very short-lived. Often, sufferers will have a family or personal history of migraines and exhibit clinical features typical of migraine headaches: children, for example, might be nauseated or have a headache, or might want to avoid bright lights or loud noises. As the migraine abates, the child might fall asleep and find that the pain goes away. Antimigraine therapy can help relieve symptoms. The abdominal migraine is different from cyclic vomiting syndrome (CVS), which is another important condition where migraines play a role. (See chapter 18 for more information on cyclic vomiting syndrome.)

The Ultimate Goal: Returning to Normal Function

One of the extremely damaging potential side effects of irritable bowel syndrome, or any functional pain syndrome, is the loss of social function in the child. He becomes unable to leave the house because of fear of being caught in an embarrassing situation. Without treatment, he eventually will stop attending school regularly and fall behind in his studies, adding yet another layer of worry and compounding the social problem.

ACTIVITY VS. AVOIDANCE

The idea that we should not use an organ or appendage that hurts in order to reduce the risk of further injury does not apply to functional pain syndromes. Avoiding use of the gut or curtailing social activities on account of the pain only causes further dysfunction. In fibromyalgia and other chronic joint syndromes, for example, intensive physical rehabilitation has been found to offer the best chances of success while pain avoidance results in weakness and, in extreme cases, the sad picture of wheelchair-bound teenagers in the prime of their lives.

In extreme cases, a debilitating vicious cycle ensues, one that is recognized clinically as recurrent abdominal pain with social disability or persistent abdominal pain syndrome with social disability (PADS). The disability becomes an intrinsic part of the problem, as the child loses peer interaction and becomes afraid of going back to school and falls further behind his peers socially and academically.

The social consequences for the older child with bellyaches who gets into this cycle can be demoralizing. Parents can help by being compassionate at all times and never doubting the child's pain, but also firmly emphasizing the importance of the prompt return to more normal function. Get your child out of the house; when at home, limit television and electronic-game playing. Additionally, parents need to speak with their child's teachers, make arrangements with the school to address time and content missed as well as concerns related to illness, and modify the child's schedule. They can give the child more leeway, but they should push ahead. It is essential that they don't render the child an invalid.

SIX STEPS TO HELP YOUR CHILD RETURN TO SCHOOL*

1. Identify and address obstacles to attendance (makeup work, for example)
2. Identify a manageable goal for school attendance, such as half days for the first week
3. Identify rewards that a child values and are within the family budget (going to a movie, a new book, an extra hour of TV)
4. Establish a schedule of rewards for school attendance
5. With your doctor's help, design a chart to track progress
6. Schedule follow-up appointments or telephone calls with the doc-

---

*Adapted from Lynn Walker, "Behavioral Management of Functional Pain," paper presented at the proceedings of the Ninth Annual Postgraduate Course, North American Society for Pediatric Gastroenterology, Hepatology and Nutrition, Orlando, Florida, October 24, 2002.

tor and school to review progress and modify the reward program as appropriate

If the situation goes on for months, then other stressors will come into play: "How can I go back to school? I've already missed weeks of course work"; "I'm going to be behind—I'm not going to be able to keep up my grades"; "Nobody believes I am sick" may all be cited as concerns. To avert this possibility, it is important to make arrangements early, think ahead, and avoid disability at all costs.

Our scientific understanding of gut hypersensitivity is in its infancy, but what we do know helps explain the puzzling complaints experienced by our patients with irritable bowel syndrome and other functional complaints. More and more, research into the origins of functional pains are shedding light and providing insight into the fundamental nature of the brain-gut communication and the adaptations we make to handle chronic pain.

Effective therapies will continue to be developed, and we can expect to see new medications targeting specific pain receptors becoming available in the coming years. Furthermore, fostering effective coping techniques based on our understanding that communication between the brain and the gut travels in both directions will translate into methods of blocking pain in the gut by tapping emotional resources. So, in the absence of a "cure," you and your child should focus on the practical steps that can be taken on a daily basis to contain the impact of pain on his development.

CHAPTER 5

Digestive Detective: Diagnostic Gastrointestinal Tests

One of the most spectacular areas of medical progress in recent years has been the increasing number of technologies available to investigate disorders of the gastrointestinal (GI) system and reach diagnoses. In some situations, we are almost on a level with *Star Trek*'s Dr. McCoy in our sophistication, but for the most part we still rely on technologies that he would, no doubt, consider primitive: blood tests, X-rays, endoscopies, nuclear scans, and magnetic resonance imaging.

Reaching a diagnosis is always the result of sifting through the wide range of possibilities suggested by the patient's history and finding evidence that either confirms or denies whatever suspicions the doctor may have. Like a detective, the doctor must sift through clues until he finds a likely suspect to pursue. Diagnostic tests are a crucial tool in getting to the bottom of a problem. At the same time, though, they often sound alarming to a parent who does not know exactly what's involved.

In this chapter, we will describe the most common medical tests used to diagnose digestive ailments so you'll know what to expect when your child is scheduled for an X-ray, an endoscopy, or a CT (computerized tomography) scan. If you are familiar with these and other related procedures, you will be in a better position to reassure your child that everything's going to be okay, because you can then talk about what the procedure involves and how long it will last. For the test to have the best chance of success, the patient should be properly prepared. If the test calls for fasting, for example, then the requirements need to be carefully followed, and you as a parent are in the best position to make sure that that happens for your child.

The information we provide does not apply in every circumstance. The duration of a particular test may differ, for example, in which case the radiologist you are working with will be able to tell you exactly what is involved with your child's specific procedure. And as always, you should consult your physician with any additional questions you may have.

X-Rays

The simplest way to visualize the intestines is to get X-ray films, which in fact can tell us a lot. Air on an X-ray film looks dark. When the intestinal-gas pattern is normal, we see air extending all the way to the large intestine. We can see not only whether it is distributed evenly, but also if the loops of intestine are dilated or full of fluid, a sign that something, such as an obstruction, is preventing the normal passage of fluid and air. A plain X-ray film can also tell us about the presence of stool in the large intestine, where it is in the colon, and whether the amounts are excessive.

Kidneys, Ureters, and Bladder (KUB), or "Flat Plate," X-Ray Film

WHAT THE TEST IS　　A few X-ray films taken while lying down under a camera.

DURATION OF TEST　　A few minutes.

DIAGNOSTIC PURPOSE(S)　　To visualize the distribution of air, fluid, and stool in the GI tract. To determine the presence of calcium deposits.

PREPARATION　　None needed.

WHAT TO TELL YOUR CHILD　　*You will lie down under a camera while they take some pictures. The test does not hurt at all. It will only take a few minutes. It will help the doctors find out what's wrong.*

Upper GI Series

When we want to visualize the digestive tract from the esophagus through the stomach and into the beginning of small intestine, we ask for a test called an upper GI series. "Series" in this case means that a number of pictures are taken. The X-ray camera used for this test is called a fluoroscope and it is almost like a video in that it allows us to see things as they are happening. Parents shouldn't be worried about the level of radiation exposure, which is well below the tolerated allowances for safety. Furthermore, the gonads are always covered with a lead apron for additional protection, because radiation is cumulative and no one needs to be exposed unnecessarily.

The first step in an upper GI series is for the baby or child to drink a white chalky liquid containing barium, a dense mineral that absorbs the X-rays and shows up as white on X-ray film, allowing doctors to see the inside of the digestive tract.

Barium is inert and nontoxic, and it is safe because it doesn't get absorbed by the body at all. It can be mixed in different consistencies, from thin to thick, and in flavors, including chocolate and strawberry, making it more drinkable. Also, upper GI procedures are timed to coincide with when the baby is due for a bottle, so babies and toddlers are more likely to drink eagerly. In older children, the test is scheduled to follow an overnight fast.

Upper GI Series

WHAT THE TEST IS   A way of looking at how food is propelled from the mouth into the stomach and just beyond, using barium and X-ray pictures.

DURATION OF TEST   About thirty minutes.

DIAGNOSTIC PURPOSE(S)   To visualize the esophagus, stomach, and duodenum.

PREPARATION   Fasting followed by ingestion of barium solution.

WHAT TO TELL YOUR CHILD   *They will take some pictures while you drink this white, chalky drink. It doesn't hurt, and all you have to do is follow the doctor's instructions when she asks you to drink or stop drinking.*

Small Bowel Follow-Through

A small bowel follow-through entails taking snapshots of barium as it moves along the digestive tract, so that the whole of the small intestine is visualized. Every half hour or so, an X-ray film is taken to track the progress of barium through the small bowel. It is commonly used for the diagnosis of conditions affecting the end of the small intestine, such as Crohn's disease.

Small Bowel Follow-Through

WHAT THE TEST IS   A series of X-ray films taken to observe the passage of barium through the small bowel.

DURATION OF TEST   Usually two to three hours, depending on how quickly the barium progresses.

DIAGNOSTIC PURPOSE(S)   To visualize the whole small bowel and identify possible areas of narrowing, inflammation, or obstruction.

PREPARATION   Fasting overnight, drinking a barium solution, waiting in the radiology department between X-ray pictures.

WHAT TO TELL YOUR CHILD   *This is going to take a while, but the doctors want to see all of your intestines. Toward the end, they will use a small paddle to put pressure over the lower part of your intestine. This is not a painful test.*

Modified Barium Swallow

Similar to the small bowel follow-through, the modified barium swallow looks only at the process of drinking. It is a test primarily for children with feeding difficulties and provides important information about what is happening to food before and after it is swallowed.

Modified Barium Swallow

WHAT THE TEST IS   A videotaped examination of the swallowing mechanism.

DURATION OF TEST   Forty-five to sixty minutes.

DIAGNOSTIC PURPOSE(S)   To visualize the swallowing mechanism and determine whether there is spilling of the food into the airway or abnormal propulsion of the food into the esophagus.

PREPARATION The child will be fasting for four to six hours, depending on age, and will be placed in a special chair while the films are taken.

WHAT TO TELL YOUR CHILD *You will be sitting up while they give you different things to drink or take from a spoon. It is very important that you cooperate so that we can find out what is happening.*

Barium Enema

A barium enema is used to identify areas of inflammation or narrowing, or the presence of polyps or other lesions, in the large intestine. Barium is introduced using a small catheter placed in the anus. The radiologist watches to ensure that the barium goes in slowly and does not escape as the position of the patient is changed to allow the solution to move along the colon.

Barium Enema

WHAT THE TEST IS X-ray films taken while barium is dripped into the colon through the rectum.

DURATION OF TEST About thirty minutes.

DIAGNOSTIC PURPOSE(S) To visualize the large intestine or rectum and identify any areas of narrowing or inflammation, or the presence of stools; to help identify the diameter changes in the colon present in Hirschsprung's disease, a congenital condition in which some of the nerve endings of the bowel are missing.

PREPARATION Colon is cleaned of stool with a laxative (in most instances); clear-liquid diet for one day.

WHAT TO TELL YOUR CHILD   *It might be uncomfortable, but it will not last very long.*

CT (or CAT) Scan

A CT scan (also called a CAT scan) is a test that uses a specialized X-ray machine to create cross-sectional images of the body in tiny slices. (CT stands for computerized tomography, and CAT stands for computerized axial tomography, both technical terms for the system that creates the images from the individual "slices.") A CT scan gathers information about solid organs like the liver, spleen, pancreas, and kidneys and the area behind the intestines. The thickness of the wall of the intestine itself can be estimated as well. CT scans are now often used to rule out appendicitis and can be used in cases of unexplained pain or when a suspicious mass is felt during a physical examination. In the future, it may be possible to examine the colon by reconstructing it with the help of CT images in a process called virtual colonoscopy.

CT Scan

WHAT THE TEST IS   Cross-sectional X-ray films of any part of the body.

DURATION OF TEST   The actual test lasts less than a minute. At least one hour of preparation should be anticipated while drinking oral contrast, a dilute form of barium that helps visualize the internal organs.

DIAGNOSTIC PURPOSE(S)   To examine the intestines, solid organs (liver, spleen, pancreas, and kidneys), and surrounding structures.

PREPARATION Drink a light barium solution in juice; sometimes may involve placement of an IV before the test.

WHAT TO TELL YOUR CHILD *You will drink a container of juice to help the doctor see the intestine. They might place an IV just before the test. This might hurt a bit, but it will be removed right after the test.*

Magnetic Resonance Imaging Test (MRI)

A magnetic resonance imaging (MRI) test does not involve the use of X-rays; instead, it uses a very large magnet and radio waves. The magnet makes all the body's molecules electrically align in one direction, at which point they are hit with a radio signal. The way the signal responds in this magnetic field depends on the amount of water in the tissues. Because each tissue contains different amounts of water, different relaxation curves are obtained, and these are used to create an image.

Among the benefits of MRIs is that with them doctors can diagnose conditions in children without having to subject them to invasive procedures. However, in contrast to CT scans, MRIs are slow, taking close to an hour to gather all the information for a study. Because any kind of motion will blur the images, it is important that the child remains motionless for the duration of the test. Consequently, most MRIs in children need to be performed while the children are under sedation or anesthesia.

Magnetic Resonance Imaging

WHAT THE TEST IS It is a special way of obtaining very precise images of the solid organs, bones, joints, and muscles, as well as the brain. In special MRIs called magnetic resonance cholan-giopancreatography (MRCP), clear images of the bile ducts, gallbladder, and pancreatic ducts can be obtained.

DURATION OF TEST   About one hour.

DIAGNOSTIC PURPOSE(S)   To examine the brain or the solid organs.

PREPARATION   Fasting, usually for six to twelve hours, to accommodate sedation or anesthesia.

WHAT TO TELL YOUR CHILD   *You will be asleep for this test, but you might hear banging noises while you are in the special machine. The test is not painful, and it will be very useful to the doctor.*

Ultrasound

Ultrasound is one of the most widely used diagnostic tests in a doctor's arsenal. It is noninvasive and involves no radiation.

Ultrasound is very sensitive and useful in identifying kidney and gallbladder stones, and distension of ducts in the liver or the ureters in the kidneys. It is also a major diagnostic tool in cardiology, as all the chambers of the heart can be identified and the blood pressure differences measured when there are heart defects. In addition, prenatal ultrasound has enabled identification of heart, spine, and brain defects as well as aided in confirming the presence of kidney obstruction and other important structural details.

Ultrasound is commonly referred to as the "jelly on the belly" test because of the conductive jelly spread over the area in question and used to "listen" to the echoed sound waves. The test is not uncomfortable, although some children will cry when pressure is applied with the lubricated probe.

Ultrasound

WHAT THE TEST IS   Imaging using high-frequency sound waves.

DURATION OF TEST   Thirty to forty minutes.

DIAGNOSTIC PURPOSE(S)   To visualize the internal organs and what surrounds them. To look for stones in the kidney or gallbladder. To determine whether the bile or pancreatic ducts are dilated. To identify cysts or free fluid in the abdomen. To examine blood flow through arteries and veins.

PREPARATION   None usually needed. When the bladder is being studied, the patient is asked to drink one to two glasses of water or juice to make it fill with urine.

WHAT TO TELL YOUR CHILD   *You will lie down in bed and the technician (or doctor) will rub your belly with some warm jelly to help her look inside. This is not a painful test, and I will be with you all the time. It should not take too long.*

Nuclear-Medicine Tests

Nuclear-medicine tests tell us how the organs, such as the liver, gall-bladder, or the stomach, function. The tests involve the injection or ingestion of extremely small amounts of radioactive chemicals. From the low levels of radiation given off by the chemicals, images can be obtained of the various parts of the body. Nuclear-medicine tests are very useful for a number of things, including identifying the site of bleeding, the flow of bile out of the liver, and even how fast the stomach empties after eating a solid or a liquid meal.

Nuclear-Medicine Tests

WHAT THE TEST IS   Imaging using special chemicals that give off low-level radiation.

DURATION OF TEST   Depends on the test, but usually about one hour. Repeated scanning is sometimes used to follow the course of the GI tract.

DIAGNOSTIC PURPOSE(S)   To visualize liver and gallbladder function, the rate of stomach emptying, the presence of inflammation, the source of bleeding, and other conditions.

PREPARATION   Fasting for a few hours, if the scan is aimed at checking stomach emptying or bile flow. Otherwise, no special preparation is needed in most cases.

WHAT TO TELL YOUR CHILD   Depends on the specific test. In cases where the chemical is given intravenously: *You will get a needle in your arm and afterward you will lie down under the camera while pictures are taken. This may take an hour, and it's important that you don't move so we get clear pictures.* (In other cases, such as GI imaging, intravenously introduced isotopes are usually used.)

Endoscopy and Colonoscopy

The upper endoscopy is a test done to visualize the inside of the digestive tract from the mouth to the second part of the duodenum. At the other end, the colonoscopy allows us to see throughout the large intestine and sometimes also the end of the small intestine, which is called the terminal ileum. Endoscopic instruments have been refined tremendously in the last few years. Today's video chips can deliver high-resolution images, as beautifully sharp as those from the best digital cameras.

With colonoscopies, the preparation for the test is usually harder than the test itself. Your child must drink a flavored but slightly salty preparation the day before, which will help to flush the colon clean. This can take several hours, and kids (not to mention adults) hate having to drink so much during such a short period of time, as it makes them feel bloated and sometimes nauseated. Also, an enema often needs to be given the morning of the procedure.

Upper Endoscopy and Colonoscopy

WHAT THE TEST IS   A direct view of the inside of the digestive tract obtained by using a video endoscope, a slender, maneuverable tube with a high-quality video chip at its end.

DURATION OF TEST   About forty-five minutes. The actual endoscopy usually takes twenty minutes; the remainder of the time is used for sedating or anesthetizing the patient.

DIAGNOSTIC PURPOSE(S)   To examine the upper or lower intestines, to obtain biopsies, and to determine the source of, and help control, bleeding.

PREPARATION   For upper endoscopy, fasting overnight. For colonoscopy, clear-liquid diet for one day and laxative regimen as prescribed by the gastroenterologist.

WHAT TO TELL YOUR CHILD   *You will be asleep during the test. When you wake up, you might feel gassy, but the gassiness should not last too long.*

Sigmoidoscopy

A sigmoidoscopy is a very limited colonoscopy that is performed when we are interested in how the lining in the lower colon

looks or when searching for the source of bright-red blood passing through the rectum. It is usually done with just one enema
preparation, and, because the procedure is quick enough and
mostly painless, we usually do not need to sedate the child. (If
cooperation is impossible, however, the procedure is scheduled
so that sedation can be administered.)

Sigmoidoscopy

WHAT THE TEST IS   A direct visualization of the lower large
intestine.

DURATION OF TEST   About fifteen minutes.

DIAGNOSTIC PURPOSE(S)   To identify possible sources of
bleeding or extent of inflammation.

PREPARATION   Generally, an enema just before the test, but
sometimes no preparation is needed.

WHAT TO TELL YOUR CHILD   *You will lie down on your side
and the doctor will look inside your bottom with a small flexible tube.
If you want, you can see what's going on by watching a TV monitor—it's kind of cool.*

Laparoscopy

This is a surgical procedure in which various instruments are
introduced through small incisions and used to identify and treat
a whole host of conditions. A small incision is made at the
umbilicus, or belly button, and in two or three other locations in
the abdomen, and through them instruments such as small scis-
sors, forceps, and even needle and thread are introduced. Using
these instruments, the surgeon is able to grasp, cut, stitch, staple,
and remove as necessary in the abdominal cavity. In general,

patients recover and return to their usual activities faster after laparoscopic surgery than they would after standard open-abdominal surgery.

Laparoscopy

WHAT THE TEST IS   A surgical procedure using special instruments introduced through small incisions in the abdominal wall, without the need for a standard, open incision.

DURATION OF TEST   Variable, depends on the problem and what needs to be done to correct it.

DIAGNOSTIC PURPOSE(S)   In cases where the test is used for diagnosis, the procedure allows direct visual inspection of the internal organs. If something abnormal is found, the surgeon can take care of it at the same time.

PREPARATION   The patient fasts for six to twelve hours, and the procedure is carried out under general anesthesia.

WHAT TO TELL YOUR CHILD   *You will have an operation to help cure your problem, and you will recover quickly. If you have pain after it's over, tell us, and the doctors will give you as much pain medicine as you need to be comfortable.*

Rectal Exam

A lot of parents and doctors think of rectal examinations as intrusive tests. When it's done with proper attention to the child, with sensitivity and gentleness, however, it does not have to be painful or embarrassing. You have to explain to the child what's to be done, position the child gently on his or her left side, and talk through the whole procedure.

The actual test may take no more than ten seconds, but in

that short time we can learn important information that we would otherwise have to guess. From my perspective as a pediatric GI specialist, it can be a crucial test in the evaluation of a child with rectal pain, constipation, or bleeding: it enables me to gauge the size of the rectum, feel the sphincter tone, see if there is stool sitting where it shouldn't be, and whether there is an explanation for the bleeding, such as a fissure or a polyp. Even so, many doctors are reluctant to perform rectal exams because they feel the procedure to be intrusive and believe they can obtain much the same information with a simple X-ray.

Rectal Exam

WHAT THE TEST IS   Examination of the anus and rectum.
DURATION OF TEST   About ten seconds.
DIAGNOSTIC PURPOSE(S)   To find the cause of rectal bleeding; to assess the degree of stool backup and constipation.
PREPARATION   None needed.
WHAT TO TELL YOUR CHILD   *It might be uncomfortable, but it's quick, and it's a very important test.*

pH Probe Test

The pH probe study is probably the most useful test there is for assessing acid reflux. It uses a sensor to measure acidity in the esophagus. To perform the test, a small wire with a sensor at its tip is fed through one nostril and advanced until its tip is in the lower part of the esophagus. An X-ray of the chest is taken to confirm the location. From that point, the sensor sends information about acidity back to a recorder.

pH Probe Test

WHAT THE TEST IS A measurement of the acidity of gastric juices that reach the esophagus as a result of gastroesophageal reflux.

DURATION OF TEST Eighteen to twenty-four hours.

DIAGNOSTIC PURPOSE(S) To quantify the duration and timing of reflux episodes. To correlate reflux or acidity with symptoms such as irritability, coughing, and nighttime crying.

PREPARATION Hold feedings for three hours before the test to avoid having a full stomach should the child vomit.

WHAT TO TELL YOUR CHILD *The doctor needs to put a small wire down your nose. This is not going to be too pleasant, but once the wire is in, you should not gag too much and the discomfort will calm down.*

Lactose Breath Test

How can you tell from the breath if someone has a problem digesting lactose? Simple: from the hydrogen content in the breath! When someone has lactose intolerance, lactose is not completely absorbed in the small intestine and reaches the large intestine, where it is fermented by bacteria. This generates hydrogen, among other gases. This hydrogen is absorbed into the blood, reaches the lungs, and is exhaled. The concentrations of hydrogen can then be measured in samples of exhaled air obtained at thirty-minute intervals after administration of the test dose. Lactose intolerance will be revealed by the hydrogen levels.

Lactose Breath Test

WHAT THE TEST IS   A measure of hydrogen in exhaled air: the hydrogen is produced by bacteria in the large intestine when malabsorbed lactose reaches it and is fermented.

DURATION OF TEST   Two to three hours.

DIAGNOSTIC PURPOSE(S)   To detect lactose intolerance.

PREPARATION   Fasting six hours before the test. Drink a sweet mix of lactose in water to begin test.

WHAT TO TELL YOUR CHILD   *You may feel some cramps during or after the test, but it will go away.*

Motility Test

Motility tests aim to measure peristalsis, the coordinated contractions of the upper GI tract or the colon. They are performed routinely in only a few medical centers. The procedure involves the placement of a catheter in the digestive tract. Along its length, this catheter has various sensing ports that are filled with water constantly but at a very slow rate. When there are changes in GI-tract pressure on the outside of a port, the change is transmitted to a recording device.

Motility Test

WHAT THE TEST IS   A measure of the strength and timing of the muscle contractions of the esophagus, stomach, duodenum, or colon.

DURATION OF TEST   Esophageal manometry, about thirty minutes; antro-duodenal, three to six hours; colonic, three to six hours.

DIAGNOSTIC PURPOSE(S)   To determine whether peristalsis is normal. To measure sphincter tone in the lower esophagus.

PREPARATION   Fasting for six hours before the test.

WHAT TO TELL YOUR CHILD   *You may feel a little uncomfortable when the sensor is inserted.* (For antro-duodenal and colonic manometry, the probe is inserted during an endoscopy or colonoscopy [for more information on these procedures, see page 88–89].)

III

The Most Common Gastrointestinal Disorders

CHAPTER 6

Feeding Difficulties in Infants

ARCHING AWAY FROM THE BOTTLE . . .

LISTLESSNESS DURING FEEDS . . .

LACK OF INTEREST IN FOOD

What could be more natural and basic than eating and drinking? Infants do it instinctively and without needing any instruction. They are born with excellent survival skills and will automatically latch on to the nipple and suck for dear life. It comes easy—for most infants, that is. Some babies do not take well to feeding. Assuming for a moment that baby has a normal hunger drive, what are some of the reasons for feeding difficulties? In this chapter, I will address this frustrating problem and provide some answers. The pediatrician and the specialist face such issues regularly; the problem is not uncommon. Each caregiver will devise ways of approaching the challenge and will offer recommendations to correct the food refusal or failure to eat normally.

The Ideal Feeder

A newborn will let you know when he is hungry, and with some luck and gentle prodding, you will gradually establish the feeding routine that suits your family best. Initially, an infant will need to be fed every two to three hours; a breast-fed baby will feed at even closer intervals of perhaps one and a half to two hours. As the weeks go by, however, all infants tend to settle into a three- to four-hour routine. Babies are notoriously fickle, though, and parents should keep in mind that feeding on demand, with the freedom to stop eating when satisfied and the reassurance that food is available whenever hunger strikes, contributes to a baby's sense of happiness associated with meals, one that babies fed on very strict schedules miss.

The Difficult Feeder

For some infants, feeding is not a pleasant activity. At meals, they are fussy, tense, and unsettled. They seem hungry, yet they fight the nipple. Their schedules are difficult to establish and parents feel pushed to overcompensate, worrying that eating so little at one time does not provide their baby with nearly enough nourishment. The concern is valid, for while some of these infants will continue to gain weight adequately, others might fail to thrive and need to be looked at more carefully in order to determine whether there is a treatable reason behind their feeding difficulties.

Many parents have discovered that their fussy baby feeds best when drowsy or sleepy. We do not understand the reason for this feeding pattern; it may be that the difficult feeder seems less aware that he is being fed when in a state of semialertness and thus less aware of pain that he might be experiencing from such issues as acid reflux or a protein allergy. Is that what's happening? Does feeding cause pain? Is swallowing accompanied by spasm of the esophagus or the stomach? Do the gums hurt? It is a very frustrating experience for parent and baby alike. Still, some difficulties may be due to physical and other barriers interfering with the natural progress of food through the digestive tract, some of which parents can easily correct.

Six Components of a Successful Meal

1. A good seal between the lips and the nipple
2. Coordinated sucking and swallowing actions
3. Effective conduct of food down the esophagus
4. Processing of food in the stomach
5. Digesting the food
6. Signaling the brain for the next meal

Usually, all the above actions happen naturally and instinctively, but when any do not, there are a variety of reasons why. The right diagnosis is key to the appropriate treatment, so let's review each of these six keys to successful feeding and explain some of the conditions impeding them and how those conditions can cause feeding difficulties.

I remember seeing Val, a thin and pale infant, for poor weight gain when she was three weeks old. After getting her full medical history, one detail in the description, how she fed, raised a red flag. Every time Val started to breast-feed, she seemed to gurgle, pull away, cough, and sound congested. Often she cried and seemed hungry, but refused to eat. No wonder she was not gaining weight! Her choking was explained when we ordered a chest X-ray and barium swallow: the barium trickled down from her throat into the esophagus and ended up in her lungs. She had a connection between the feeding and breathing pipes! This early diagnosis helped prevent major complications, and Val was completely well after corrective surgery.

1. A GOOD SEAL BETWEEN THE LIPS AND THE NIPPLE

CONDITION	REASON FOR UNSUCCESSFUL FEEDING
Structural problems such as a cleft lip and palate	The small chin and tongue are crowded and it is difficult to fit anything else in the mouth
Poor muscle tone	Weak muscle tone (hypotonia) can be a symptom of neurological handicap such as cerebral palsy (CP)
Hypersensitive gag reflex or sensory issues	The gag reflex is triggered whenever exposed to certain textures or food that is too cold or hot
Congenital conditions such as undeveloped and obstructed nasal passages Nasal passages clogged by allergies or reactions to environmental irritants such as cigarette smoke, dust, or mold, or by large tonsils and adenoids	Infants need to breath through the nose. It takes them a little more time to figure out that they can just as easily breathe through the mouth. As a result, any condition that induces nasal congestion will interfere with proper mouth closure.

2. COORDINATED SUCKING AND SWALLOWING ACTIONS

All the muscle groups involved in the coordinated ballet that is sucking and swallowing have to work in perfectly harmonious synchrony. As a mouthful of milk slides down the esophagus, sensors have to tell the baby the mouth is full. Failure to do so can result in any of the following:

- Overfilling: the baby's ability to manage what went into the mouth is overwhelming and the baby gags, sputters, or chokes.
- Pooling of secretions and food in the back of the throat
- Choking, coughing, and sputtering
- Regurgitation of food through the nose
- Aspiration of food into the lungs

3. EFFECTIVE CONDUCT OF FOOD DOWN THE ESOPHAGUS

Once the milk is in the esophagus, it must reach the stomach. Here are some reasons why this might not happen:

CONDITION	REASON FOR UNSUCCESSFUL FEEDING
Acid reflux or allergic reaction	The esophagus wall may become inflamed and cause painful spasm with every swallow
Congenital webs	Esophagus is narrowed, interfering with normal passage of food
Achalasia, a rare condition in which the lower sphincter does not relax normally	Food never reaches the stomach, accumulates in the esophagus, and is vomited; may also cause nighttime cough or even pneumonia.

continued on next page

CONDITION	REASON FOR UNSUCCESSFUL FEEDING
Tracheo-esophageal, or T-E, fistula: esophagus and airway (trachea) are connected	Congenital problem causes food to seep into lungs, resulting in coughing, congestion, and resistance to feeding
Foreign body in esophagus or other blockage	Esophagus may be inflamed or blocked

4. PROCESSING OF FOOD IN THE STOMACH

Infants and children with inflammation of the stomach (gastritis) will experience discomfort or pain when food reaches the stomach. Gastritis can result from protein allergies, excessive acidity in the stomach, or gastroenteritis brought on by viruses or bacteria.

Discomfort can also result from overeating or by having a stomach that is in spasm and does not relax appropriately to receive food. This latter condition is often seen in premature babies and other children in whom there are immaturities of the digestive tract. In rare cases, the discomfort can result from *pyloric stenosis,* a narrowing of the pyloric channel. This narrowing prevents food from getting into the intestine, building up the pressure in the stomach, which can lead to projectile vomiting. The problem will worsen until it is corrected surgically.

NOTE   I believe that if babies experience pain and nausea with eating, they will develop aversions to food. They become reluctant to continue eating and stop after a few swallows or bites, as if their body remembers the discomfort and sends warning signals to avoid repeating the experience.

5. DIGESTING THE FOOD

Any interference with the normal breakdown of carbohydrates, fats, and proteins can result in diarrhea, excessive gas, and pain. (For more information, review the detailed description of the digestive process provided in chapter 1.)

6. SIGNALING THE BRAIN FOR THE NEXT MEAL

This final component of the feeding process brings us back to the mysterious and extraordinary system that communicates to the baby that it is time for another meal. By now, food has been digested, absorbed, and used by the body, and almost on cue, three or four hours after the previous bottle, a cry sounds: "I need a refill!"

WHEN AN INFANT IS NOT HUNGRY

I would like to mention the rare, but very real, phenomenon of infants who don't appear ever to be hungry. This alarms parents when it occurs, and babies exhibiting this behavior remain a mystery to feeding specialists, gastroenterologists, neurologists, psychologists, and nutritionists alike. It is as if a primary instinct for survival is missing. Left to their own devices, these infants will fail to thrive or will grow very slowly. They might need more aggressive medical interventions (for example, tube feedings), and a great deal of dedication from their parents, to avoid malnutrition.

Parents of children who are poor feeders often feel as if they face this problem alone. Dealing with a child who refuses to accept the food they so lovingly offer is demoralizing and depressing. Through their health care provider or specialist, however, parents can be referred to a feeding and speech therapist who can help them overcome the feeding refusal, especially when it is aggravated by oral hypersensitivity. The visits offer an opportunity to plan feeding strategies, discuss optimal dietary recommendations, and monitor the baby's growth and development.

Hopefully, this brief overview of some of the complexities involved with successful infant feeding will help you overcome some of the frustrating stumbling blocks that can prevent that from happening.

CHAPTER 7

How to Cope with Infantile Colic

IRRITABILITY . . . INCONSOLABLE CRYING . . .
LEG KICKING

Your month-old child is irritable. She's arching her back and crying. She has what appear to be stomach cramps and is expelling an excessive amount of gas. She's pushing the breast or the bottle away and is refusing to eat. If she's managed to get anything down recently, at least some of it was regurgitated.

A child who cries inconsolably has the power to turn any household upside down. Frantic attempts to quiet a screaming baby account for a high proportion of infant injury and even death from so-called shaken-baby syndrome. Identifying colic, however, goes a long way toward managing the situation effectively and preventing frustration from boiling over. The major challenge, both for parents and health care providers, is that colic mimics other common conditions seen in young infants, especially protein allergy and gastroesophageal reflux (GER).

What Is Colic?

First and foremost, colic is not a disease. It certainly looks as though it is when screaming, pulling on the legs, and passing gas all suggest that something is really wrong with the intestines, but colic is actually a pattern of behavior shown by infants, and is an extension of normal crying—albeit a very distressing and frustrating extension, to be sure.

The Rule of Threes, proposed by Dr. Marc Weissbluth in 1958, is still widely accepted as a working definition of colic. In Dr. Weissbluth's formulation, an infant's inconsolable crying may be deemed colic if it starts after three weeks of age, lasts for more than three hours a day, and occurs at least three times a week for more than three weeks (weeks need not be consecutive). Further criteria for colic include no physical cause for the crying and apparent health in every respect.

The vast majority of babies stop displaying colic symptoms around the age of three months. In around 10 percent of infants, however, colic will continue—to everyone's despair.

RESEARCH ON CRYING

Research indicates that hunger accounts for about one-third of infant crying episodes, while wet or soiled diapers explain about 20 percent. Amazingly, the studies indicate that no explanation could be found for almost 30 percent of the crying episodes: babies just cry. It is a form of communication: when they're tired, when they're overwhelmed, or perhaps because they can't yet tell us what they are feeling in words.

Studies at the Mayo Clinic note that most children cry for anywhere from one to eleven minutes per hour. The minimum observed was forty-eight minutes per day, which works out to just two minutes an hour. The maximum was four hours. Colic represents excessive normal crying.

What Causes Colic?

We still don't know for sure what causes colic. Proposed explanations cite hormonal imbalances, immature neurotransmitters in the brain and gut, and even temperament: babies who are colicky have been variously described as vigorous, intense, excitable, and easily startled. Current research suggests that colic is a manifestation of disrupted sleep patterns and related to overload of the baby's immature sensory system.

Because a child's gastrointestinal tract is immature, it is hard to know if there is a digestive reason for the excessive crying. Sometimes reflux is suspected, but endoscopy will often reveal no evidence of inflammation or damage—yet the baby cries and exhibits feeding difficulties as if there were. Another explanation for colic could be that muscles in the esophagus, stomach, or intestines are in spasm, but here too there is still a lack of evidence from which to draw any definitive conclusions. More often than not, babies seem to have intestinal pain because they are crying, and not the other way around!

Some Important Characteristics of Colic

Colic remains an inexact science, but even so, there are some characteristics and components that seem to appear consistently among colicky babies. These include:

- The baby will have unexplained irritability, crying, and fretfulness
- Piercing, screaming attacks, with clenched fists and apparent abdominal pain
- Waxing and waning of symptoms: sometimes they will be intense, other times more mild—most colicky babies have good days, too
- Colic management is unpredictable—what works one day may not work the next

How to Cope with Colic

Parents need to recognize colic for what it is, that it is unexplainable and frustrating but nevertheless passing, and know they can do things to cope with their and their infant's sensory overload. It may help to remind yourself of the following:

- Your colicky baby is healthy and thriving.
- Colic will decrease. (Make this your mantra. The situation won't last forever. It won't last forever. *It won't last forever.*)
- There are no colicky one-year-olds.
- Colic is not caused by anything you have done or are doing "wrong" (no guilt!).

A lot has been written about the tense parent communicating their nervousness and frustration to their infant, and it's true that some babies are exquisitely sensitive to those vibes. That does not account for colic developing in the first place, but on the other hand, keeping calm and handling your baby with confidence will have a marked effect on her behavior (and yours!).

When colic begins, both the physician and the parents will have a hard time believing there is nothing wrong with the child. At this point, some changes in the diet may be suggested, and if reflux is suspected, using antacids for a trial period is recommended. You never know if these measures will bring some relief, and under the circumstances, even an hour (or half hour) of quiet is a welcome break.

HELPFUL HINTS: COPING WITH A COLICKY BABY

1. Get enough sleep.
2. Find a trusted friend, relative, or help to take over for a few hours.
3. Have a life. Don't let fatigue and worry overwhelm you.

When other causes for crying are ruled out and the baby's condition is pronounced colic, parents must understand that colic is not going to disappear by magic with a change in formula or the introduction of a particular medication. But also get used to the idea that this is just a developmental stage on the way to more mature sleeping patterns and reactions to sensory stimulations: you'll be able to wait it out more patiently and more positively. Anticipating the crying episodes before they happen, and changing some routines to soothe the baby's frayed nerves, can go a long way toward minimizing the impact of colic.

SHAKEN-BABY SYNDROME

Colic remains a major risk factor for shaken-baby syndrome, in which an overwhelmed and sleep-deprived parent trying to stop the crying can unwittingly shake the baby so hard as to cause neurological damage that can result in blindness, brain damage, or even death. Medical practices and support groups have active information campaigns aimed at preventing shaken-baby syndrome; some of their Web sites appear in the appendix.

HELPFUL HINTS: MANAGING COLIC

Managing colic effectively involves counteracting the over-stimulation that seems to tip infants over the edge at the end of the day. First, make sure that the baby is not hungry, wet, too cold, or too hot. Next, look around you: Are the lights too bright? Can you do anything about that noise? Do everything possible to provide a calm environment, and use some time-honored tricks to help soothe the baby:

- Repetitive slow motion: carry or sit with baby
- Try white noise and the rumble and motion of a driving car
- Gentle massage and acupressure

Medications

Medications are not really a useful option for dealing with colic. The only one found to be effective when compared to placebo was dicyclomine, which is sold as Bentyl. However, use of this drug in young infants can be associated with side effects, and hence this medication is not routinely recommended. Over-the-counter gas medications are also popular. Simethicone drops, found in products such as Mylicon, for example, may work in some cases because they help break down large bubbles of gas. But while the idea is to help the baby pass gas more easily and with less discomfort, the fact is that no significant differences could be detected in the duration or intensity of the crying episodes when babies given simethicone were compared to those administered a placebo.

Again, remember that colic is not a disease but rather an exaggerated expression of crying and fussiness caused by immaturity and sensory overload. It's not caused by an underlying intestinal problem and does not cause any harm to the baby. Colicky babies are vivacious, high strung, and intense. They seem to be highly attuned to their environment, and that is the way they are "wired." There is nothing wrong with them; they'll get over this phase, and so will you. While it lasts, though, finding effective means of coping is very important: maintaining your balance comes first. Do not let yourself become sleep deprived or guilt ridden. Don't take colic personally!

CHAPTER 8

What Causes Reflux and Gastroesophageal Reflux Disease?

SPITTING UP . . . VOMITING . . . IRRITABILITY . . .
FOOD REFUSAL OR CRYING WHILE FEEDING . . .
CHOKING . . . NIGHTTIME COUGH OR HOARSE
VOICE

Not a day goes by in my practice without reflux being raised by some concerned parents. Why has reflux become such a concern in children? Don't all children spit up? When did spitting (or upchucking or wet burping) turn into such a hot health issue? Are we overreacting to what used to be taken for granted?

This chapter will describe the difference between "normal" reflux and a reflux problem, known as gastroesophageal reflux disease, or GERD. It will provide you with a better handle on what to do when reflux disease is suspected, how the problem can be investigated, and what new and effective means can be used to control it.

From my perspective as a pediatric gastroenterologist, parents seem to know much more about reflux today than they did five years ago. The reason may be that by the time they see a specialist like myself, their health care provider has already described the condition and tried to resolve it by modifying the diet and prescribing over-the-counter antacids. Through such exposure, reflux has become a household term.

What Causes Reflux?

Reflux describes the phenomenon of stomach contents coming back up to the mouth. Normally, the food we swallow is kept in the stomach by the lower sphincter, the ring of muscle at the end of the esophagus. This opening relaxes every time we swallow so as to let food reach the stomach in one smooth swoop, but it should not allow food back up again (for details, see chapter 1).

As we eat, the stomach fills with food and liquid as well as air we normally swallow with our food, not only increasing pressure in it but also inducing the strong muscles of the stomach to begin pushing and churning the food. If the lower sphincter relaxes, it can allow the air bubble *and* the food to come right up. Such unexpected relaxations of the sphincter are the main reason for excessive reflux in children.

In infants, overfeeding is one of the main factors that aggravate reflux. Too much food overstretches the stomach and food just surges upward. Because the esophagus is so small in infants, even a few extra tablespoons of formula will make it to the mouth, and, not infrequently, find its way out through the nose. Parents sometimes get nervous when they see formula or food come up this way, but it is nothing more serious than volume overload.

▮▮▮

Reflux of stomach contents is a normal event in infants and young children, a product of the immaturity of the esophageal muscles and the stomach, and it improves as the child begins to sit independently. This so-called physiological reflux requires only an adjustment to the feeding and position routines to minimize stomach overfilling and the resulting overflow.

Diagnosis of Persistent Reflux

When a child is experiencing reflux, we must always consider whether the amount of reflux is abnormal: is it causing problems or will the child naturally outgrow it? When recurrent symptoms (such as crying and feeding difficulties) point to irritation of the esophagus, or vomiting becomes serious enough to cause a slowdown in the child's weight gain, action must be taken. If protein allergy is the suspected cause, the pediatrician might recommend a change in formula; when the cause is undetermined, a first step might be to start the child on some antireflux medications or refer the baby for evaluation by a specialist, who can decide whether any diagnostic tests may be needed to see if acid is reaching the esophagus and causing irritation. (See chapter 5 for descriptions of common diagnostic tests.)

Some infants and toddlers with significant acid reflux do not spit up much—the amounts are small enough to be reswallowed—and in such cases we do not know if damage is being done to the esophagus in the form of esophagitis, an inflammation of the esophagus. They are called silent refluxers, and sometimes their chronic cough, asthma, or even hoarseness are due to the constant exposure to acid, and reflux must be treated.

Treatment of Reflux

Treatment of reflux can begin at home. There are some foods that might promote or aggravate reflux in children, and they should be avoided. Among these are caffeinated sodas, chocolate and peppermint, and spicy, acidic, fried, and fatty foods. Eating within two or three hours of going to bed should also be avoided. Such simple measures can go a long way in relieving reflux.

If the situation is more serious, medical management of reflux aims at suppressing acidity, and a whole array of products are available. If the reflux is mild and temporary relief is necessary, a liquid over-the-counter antacid like Maalox or Mylanta, or a coating type of foaming agent like Gaviscon (sodium alginate) can be used. Gaviscon has surface characteristics different from other coating agents; these seem to help it stick to the lining of the esophagus longer than the others, but it is not as strong an acid suppressant as the Maalox- and Mylanta-style preparations. When a more long-lasting acid suppression is required, products like Zantac, Pepcid, Prevacid, Prilosec, Nexium, and others can be used. These medications are prescribed by your health care provider or gastroenterologist.

PYLORIC STENOSIS

The muscles of the pylorus, the sphincter between the stomach and duodenum, are normally paper-thin. When they relax, there is a nice wide-open channel, and food flows easily through it. In cases of pyloric stenosis, the situation is very different: "stenosis" means "narrowing," and that is exactly what happens to the channel when the muscles become thickened. The muscle can expand so much that there is no room left for food to get out, essentially forming an obstruction.

Pyloric stenosis occurs in 1 of every 4,000 births, most commonly in firstborn males. The thickening does not happen at birth, but rather develops over the first six weeks of life (though sometimes later). When the stomach has no functioning exit, its contractions, as it tries to empty, are all directed upward, and the result is an especially forceful form of vomiting known as *projectile vomiting*. Food will shoot out with force, like a geyser, landing two to three feet away, much to the parent's astonishment and alarm. Pyloric stenosis is corrected surgically, and the prognosis for complete recovery is excellent.

Gastroesophageal Reflux Disease

As alluded to at the beginning of this chapter, the distinction between reflux and reflux disease is a crucial one. Fortunately, while practically every newborn refluxes, only a small number of children have reflux disease. We define reflux disease, or pathological reflux, as reflux that results in impaired growth due to excessive loss of nutrients, feeding difficulties, irritability, or other significant health concerns traceable to the reflux.

For example, infants with reflux disease might fail to grow because they simply cannot bring themselves to eat enough because it hurts too much, or they eat but lose more than they actually keep down. Other children will resist eating and cry excessively, either because the acidity bothers them (an adult would describe the feeling as heartburn), or because they experience pain in the esophagus: an inflamed esophagus does not work well and might cause muscle spasms. Another problem associated with reflux is that when the acid washes against the lining of the esophagus for too long, ulcers can develop, and not only do they hurt, but in some instances they bleed slowly and might bring on anemia or iron deficiency. For all of these reasons, reflux disease deserves an evaluation by a gastrointestinal specialist and management with available and effective strategies for resolving the damaging effects of acid.

In many children, though, the warning signs of reflux are more subtle and therefore more difficult to detect. A few symptoms to keep in mind include: a nighttime cough that does not appear to accompany a cold, a chronic cold that lasts for weeks but does not seem to be from a virus, an unexplained hoarse voice, and difficult-to-control asthma. Should a child exhibit any of these symptoms, reflux may be the cause. However, as these symptoms make clear, reflux disease can imitate many conditions. Therefore, pinpointing the real reason might take some detective work, medication, or dietary changes, and if necessary, diagnostic tests. The good news is that we have the tools to treat this disease effectively.

REFLUX DISEASE IN THE NEUROLOGICALLY IMPAIRED CHILD

Children with cerebral palsy and other neurologically debilitating conditions are at a particularly high risk for reflux disease. They often suffer from excessive muscle tone in certain muscle groups and low tone in others. As a result, they have trouble handling their own secretions, choking frequently, retching, and gagging. With each gag, the pressure in the stomach increases, causing reflux. Children with seizures and children with progressive nervous-system disorders will often have discoordination of their stomach emptying, in which the relaxation of the pylorus does not occur at the same time that the stomach is trying to empty itself. The resulting pressure can trigger reflux. If acid exposure is excessive, ulcers in the esophagus might progress to scars and narrowing.

Happy Spitters

"Doctor, you have to do something! It's impossible to keep cleaning after her all day long! The carpets are one big stain, and so is the sofa, and don't ask about the dry cleaning bills!" Behind all this agitation was Monique, a calm, sweet three-month-old, a content child already flashing a social smile and showing a hearty appetite. She breast-fed eagerly and efficiently and was thriving beautifully—all the while consistently spitting up large mouthfuls, usually within a half hour of eating. As I watched her being burped, two things impressed me the most: she simply opened her mouth and milk dribbled out of her chin, and she was in no distress or pain. As such, Monique was a typical "happy spitter": her wet burps reflected a full tummy and overflow, and no reflux disease. She had no discomfort, because milk does not irritate the lining of the esophagus or the throat, and she continued to gain weight because she was eating plenty, if a little too much for her stomach's capacity.

Being able to reassure her parents, having them focus on how well she was developing, and telling them that her spitting up would resolve on its own by the time she started sitting up—most babies will simply stop doing it in due time, more than 75 percent of them by the time they start sitting by themselves at six months or so.

Managing the happy spitter involves a combination of changes in the feeding routine and what we like to call "tincture of time": simply being patient and understanding what is going on and how it will resolve itself at the end. Recommended changes include the following:

• **Thickening feedings:**   Adding rice cereal—one tablespoon of rice cereal per ounce of formula—might decrease the number of times a baby spits up and might also help with fussiness and crying. (If rice cereal is added to formula, the bottle's nipple might need to be widened to allow sufficient flow.)

• **Frequent small feedings:**   Some babies spit up because they swallow a lot of air when they feed. Small feedings every two to three hours might help to minimize the overstretching of the stomach caused by air intake. Babies should be burped often during feeding to get rid of any excess air.

• **Sit up:**   The baby should be held in an upright position on a parent's lap during feeding, and kept in this position, or in a stroller or appropriate infant seat, for thirty minutes afterward. The chest should be positioned above the belly and the back ought to be straight: it is important that the baby does not slump when sitting because that will put pressure on the stomach. Babies tend to slump or slouch if they are in a high chair, walker, or car seat, which is why these are not recommended resting places to use for a baby after a feed.

Reflux in the Infant with Apparent Life-Threatening Events

Apparent life-threatening events (ALTEs) are frightening episodes in which young infants suddenly turn pale or blue and struggle briefly before going limp and seemingly lifeless. ALTEs need to be evaluated thoroughly in a medical facility, as they can be a manifestation of serious problems such as infection, cardiac disease, or neurological abnormalities. The possibility of reflux as a possible cause is considered only after these other conditions have been ruled out by a battery of tests.

A detailed history will elicit important information, clarifying the sequence of events and the possible connection between reflux and the episode. For example, many parents will tell how they had just fed their child before putting her down for a diaper change when she just went blue and limp, or they might describe hearing gurgling sounds before the episode. Such information is essential, because in these cases, it suggests the mechanism of the ALTE: formula has refluxed and reached the throat. The upper airway, sensing the presence of liquid there, closes off in order to prevent the formula from aspirating, or going into the lungs. This closing up is accompanied by the body movements of the child struggling to breathe, after which the whole body relaxes and goes limp. Parents often use mouth-to-mouth resuscitation and chest compressions when confronted with this frightening situation.

Fortunately, in many cases, children recover and look perfectly fine by the time they are brought to the emergency room, while parents are usually very relieved but puzzled and frightened at the same time. Lifestyle changes—such as upright positioning after meals, frequent burping, and small-volume feeding—and other antireflux measures will minimize the chances of any ALTEs in the future.

CHAPTER 9

The Causes of Intestinal Gas
and the Low-Gas Diet

GULPING . . . BURPING . . . FLATULENCE

Everyone has gas in his or her digestive tract, and, in fact, when we look at an X-ray film of a child's intestines, it is always reassuring to see air throughout. It tells us that the system is open from top to bottom and that the intestine is not blocked anywhere along the way.

Intestinal gas comes from two main sources: swallowed air and normal chemical reactions that take place in the large intestine when undigested food is broken down by bacteria. For the most part, gas leaves the intestine without causing any discomfort. It is either expelled from the mouth by belches or burps, or through the rectum as flatus.

It's clear that different people generate different kinds and amounts of gas. What seems excessive to one person might in fact still be absolutely normal for another, but most of us will produce from one to three pints a day and pass gas about fourteen to twenty-three times a day. (How's that for a fascinating trivia question?) Gas becomes a problem when the intestine stretches excessively or when the sensitivity for pain is enhanced, as it is in irritable bowel syndrome.

Swallowed Air

The mere process of being alive—talking, crying, and eating—results in air being swallowed. With every gulp, a baby takes in approximately three-quarters to one teaspoon of air. Collapsible milk bottles with special nipples have been devised to reduce the amount of ingested air, but it's not really possible to drink milk or formula from a bottle or cup without swallowing a certain amount of air.

A baby is actually born with no air in the intestine. Within an hour or so after her first cry, though, the air she has swallowed reaches the colon. If there is a narrowing (stenosis) or an obstruction (atresia) anywhere along the way, a bottleneck will be created and the baby will suffer from crampy pain and nausea as the intestine tries to push the air through. Normally, however, air is expelled easily and in most babies, swallowing air causes no major problems. Some babies, especially those who eat too quickly or those with latching problems (see chapter 6), are more likely to gulp when they are fed. These gulpers need to be burped more often to avoid the discomfort that comes with reflux or distension caused by too much air inside.

Some children, in fact, swallow so much air that they need to see the doctor because they develop an extremely big belly. Their abdomens are so bloated that their clothes have to be loosened. Reassuringly, when an X-ray film is taken, all we see is gas throughout the bowel. And even with these excessive amounts of swelling, the child is not particularly uncomfortable. The gas moves smoothly, without producing cramps. When examined, the belly is hypertympanic, which means, literally, like a drum. The presence of such abdominal distension always raises concern about the possibility of an underlying tumor, enlargement of the liver, spleen or other organs, or a blockage.

Activities like intentionally swallowing air and making shockingly loud belches should be discouraged. They can actually be habit forming, and such behavior is hard to modify. I can remember a good number of patients (usually teenagers) whose main complaint was uncontrollable loud belching. Sure, this can be a sign of reflux, dyspepsia, or hyperacidity, but when someone can belch every five minutes, as they often demonstrate readily in the office, we can safely conclude that they're swallowing air. We simply do not manufacture that volume of air at such short intervals.

Gas from Food

Some food products are not digested in the small intestine because enzymes that would normally break them down are either absent or work inefficiently. Once this undigested food reaches the colon, bacteria will break it down, producing a variety of gases as by-products.

THE MOST COMMON GAS-PRODUCING FOODS

• **Lactose**   Lactose is the sugar found in milk and milk products such as cheese, cream, and ice cream. It is also in many processed foods. Lactose intolerance is common, especially in people of African, Native American, or Asian descent. (Lactose intolerance is discussed in detail in chapter 10.)

• **Sorbitol**   Sorbitol is a specific type of sugar found in apples, pears, peaches, and prunes, and it is used as a sweetener in sugar-free candy and chewing gum. (See chapter 12 on diarrhea for more on sorbitol.)

• **Raffinose and stachyose**   Found in beans, lentils, peas, and, in much smaller amounts, in vegetables like cabbage, broccoli, and cauliflower, raffinose and stachyose are complex sugars for which humans lack the enzyme to break down.

• **Fiber**   Soluble fiber in oat bran, beans, peas, and fruit produces gas when it is broken down in the large intestine.

THE LOW-GAS DIET

When starting a low-gas diet, a number of foods, especially raw vegetables, should be avoided completely. Within a few days, there will be a noticeable difference in the frequency and intensity of the gas passed. Once the effect of the low-gas diet is felt and an improvement in gas-related pain and other complaints is noticed, small amounts of any of these "forbidden" foods can be reintroduced.

It is important that only one item at a time should be reintroduced—and then, very gradually. Fiber, especially, must be handled with care. When fiber is introduced too quickly to a low-gas diet, the volume of gas produced will increase markedly. The intestine will not be able to adapt immediately to the high volume of gas, and pain could result. So, again, the recommendation is to introduce it in small amounts.

FOODS TO AVOID IN A LOW-GAS DIET

- Complex fiber, as that in multigrain cereals
- Raw, crunchy vegetables such as broccoli, cauliflower, string beans, peas, and cabbage
- Cucumbers and pickles
- Asparagus
- Artichokes
- Onions
- Tomato and other sauces made with an onion base
- Undercooked ("al dente") pasta
- Doughy bagels (less gassy when toasted)
- Dry fruits (especially apricots, figs, apples, and prunes)
- Chewy candy

HYDROGEN, CARBON DIOXIDE, AND . . . METHANE?!

As mentioned, different people generate different kinds and different amounts of gas. Interestingly, many of these differences are genetically determined. There are over two hundred gases in flatus, many only in trace amounts. Most people (95 percent) generate hydrogen and carbon dioxide, neither of which has any odor. Flatus owes its bad smell to trace amounts of gases that contain sulfur derivatives and other chemicals whose presence and concentrations result from our genes and the bacteria living in our guts. The intestines of one-third of the population, for example, produce methane gas. Bacteria might not be a factor only in gas: there's been a lot of interest in the theory that colon cancer is somehow related to the bacterial flora some people have and the bacteria's tendency to generate carcinogenic chemicals to which the lining of the colon is exposed.

Gas Pain in Infants

When a baby is crying, many parents assume that it's gas. We know, however, that children can cry for a number of reasons, and also that screaming children will compress their stomach and large intestine and expel whatever gas has accumulated there. So, when you hear the gas being expelled, don't assume that it was the reason for the pain. After all, when a child with an ear infection screams and gulps excessively, he'll also pass gas, not because of intestinal discomfort, but because the earache is making him cry.

The golden rule for the management of excessive gas is prevention or avoidance of the foodstuff or the activities that cause it to accumulate. Even so, if a child passes a lot of gas and is perfectly content, then there is no reason to change his diet and specifically avoid gas-producing foods. There is a positive benefit in continuing to eat these healthy cereals, fruits, and vegetables, and in any case, the colonic bacteria adapts to them with time.

Treatment

If treatment for gas is desired, over-the-counter medicines can help with some disorders that cause gas. Adding a product containing the enzyme lactase to milk or chewing a lactase tablet, for example, can help the lactose intolerant. (Of course, lactose-reduced milk is also available.) Similarly, the enzyme sucrase can be taken in tablet form to help digest and decrease gas brought on by sugar in certain fruits and juices.

None of the over-the-counter anti-gas preparations are particularly effective in decreasing excessive gas. About the best that can be done is to use antacids containing simethicone, which joins gas bubbles together in the stomach making them easier to expel, but these products are not effective in countering gas generated in the colon. For older children or teenagers, charcoal tablets (such as Charcocaps) may help with gas in the colon when taken just before and just after a meal, but don't count on dramatic results.

Although intestinal gas can be painful, embarrassing, or a source of concern, in most cases a careful review of the diet will go a long way toward identifying possible culprits and helping you take the necessary steps to minimize the discomfort. In the case of the air swallower, behavior modification and self-awareness will assist in resolving the problem. Sometimes this is easier said than done, but the challenge can be met with consistency and motivation.

CHAPTER 10

Understanding and Managing
Lactose Intolerance

GASSINESS . . . DIARRHEA . . .

RUMBLING AND GROWLING NOISES . . .

STOMACH CRAMPS

Lactose is the main sugar found in milk. People who are lactose intolerant are unable to digest this sugar because they have a shortage of lactase, an enzyme that when present is produced by cells that line the small intestine. This enzyme is responsible for breaking down lactose into the simpler sugars glucose and galactose. If the enzyme is in short supply, or is missing entirely, then eating or drinking anything that contains lactose can lead to symptoms such as gas or diarrhea. The enzyme can also be lost as a result of a viral infection or through a variety of other reasons such as food allergy or celiac disease. It is important to understand that symptoms of lactose intolerance can be managed with a controlled diet.

Lactose intolerance is very prevalent around the world; in the United States alone, perhaps as many as fifty million people are lactose intolerant. Some ethnic groups and populations are affected more than others: while the condition is rare among people from northern European backgrounds, up to 75 percent of African Americans, Mexican Americans, and Native Americans and 90 percent of Asian Americans are lactose intolerant.

Causes

Certain digestive diseases and injuries to the small intestine can decrease lactase production. In rare cases, a child can be born without the ability to produce lactase. However, in most people, the intolerance develops over time, for after the age of two, the body naturally produces less lactase—(teenagers produce only about 10 percent as much lactase as infants do, adults even less). Many people will not start experiencing symptoms until they are middle aged. Adult-onset lactose intolerance is genetically determined: consistent consumption of milk products will not stave it off, nor will avoidance of milk products hasten it.

Sources of Lactose

Not all sources of lactose are obvious. Milk and milk products, such as cheese, cream, cream cheese, sour cream, ice cream, and the like, are easy to identify and avoid, but lactose can be found in many prepared and processed foods. Here are just a few examples:

Bread and other baked goods

Processed breakfast cereals

Instant potatoes, soups, and hot drinks

Margarine

Nonkosher lunch meats

Salad dressings

Candies and snacks

Mixes for baked goods like pancakes, biscuits, and cookies

Milk-derived ingredients may also be included in such "nondairy" products as powdered coffee creamer. Hence, parents need to read food labels carefully and watch out for not only milk and lactose but also items like curds, whey, milk by-products, dry milk solids, and nonfat dry milk powder. These all contain some lactose.

Lactose is also found in more than 20 percent of prescription drugs and about 6 percent of over-the-counter medicines, including some tablets for stomach acid and gas. In most cases, the amounts of lactose are small enough that it won't be necessary to avoid these medications, but a pharmacist can answer questions about the amounts of lactose in various medicines.

Symptoms

Symptoms of lactose intolerance include nausea, cramps, bloating, gas, and diarrhea. These symptoms can arise from thirty minutes to two hours after eating or drinking something that contains lactose. The severity of the symptoms varies and depends on the amount of lactose an individual can tolerate.

Diagnosis

Lactose intolerance can de diagnosed by a lactose-tolerance test, a hydrogen breath test, or direct measurement of the enzyme activity in the small intestine.

HYDROGEN BREATH TEST

As the name implies, the hydrogen breath test measures the concentration of hydrogen gas in exhaled breath. Normally, very little hydrogen is detectable in the breath and elevated levels of it can indicate lactose intolerance. This is because undigested lactose in the colon is fermented by bacteria, and various gases—including hydrogen—are produced. The hydrogen is then absorbed from the intestines, carried through the bloodstream to the lungs, and exhaled. If a lot of hydrogen is exhaled, that indicates fermentation is taking place, and the next step is to see if lactose might be the cause.

To prepare for the test, the child drinks a lactose dose equivalent to twelve to twenty-five ounces of milk, and the breath is analyzed at regular intervals while symptoms of gas, cramps, or diarrhea are recorded by the parents. If the test shows elevated levels of hydrogen in the breath, then lactose intolerance can be confirmed. (Certain foods, medications, and cigarettes can affect the test's accuracy and should be avoided before taking the test.)

Because this test involves blowing air into a bag, however, some small children will have a hard time cooperating. (See chapter 5 for more details on the lactose breath test.) If lactose intolerance is suspected, the child can easily be put on a lactose-free or lactose-restricted diet, with parents observing any changes in symptoms. In other cases, if diagnosis of lactose intolerance needs to be confirmed in someone with symptoms of irritable bowel syndrome or other obscure complaints, the breath test can help us clear the issue in three hours.

Treatment

It is not possible to improve the body's ability to produce lactase, but the symptoms of lactose intolerance can be controlled by adjusting your child's diet. Young children with lactase deficiency shouldn't eat any foods that contain lactose. Older children, meanwhile, do not need to avoid lactose completely, as they differ in the amounts they can handle. (For example, a child might suffer symptoms after drinking one glass of milk but another might be able to eat ice cream and aged cheese like cheddar or parmesan, but not Swiss.) Through trial and error, you can determine what works for your child and make a list to help you feed your child and help your child cope in social situations.

For those who react to small amounts of lactose or have trouble limiting the intake of foods that contain lactose, lactase enzyme is available without a prescription in tablet form. Lactose-free and lactose-reduced milk is also available in most food stores.

CALCIUM

Milk contains calcium, which is essential for the growth and repair of bones throughout life. From the middle years on, a shortage of calcium can lead to osteoporosis, which manifests in fragile bones.

RECOMMENDED DAILY ALLOWANCE (RDA) FOR CALCIUM	
AGE	RECOMMENDED DAILY ALLOWANCE OF CALCIUM (MG PER DAY)
Birth to 5 months	400
5 months to 1 year	600
1 to 10 years	800
11 to 24 years	1,200
25 years and older	800

If milk must be avoided, other good sources of calcium include green vegetables like broccoli and kale, and fish with soft, edible bones, like salmon and sardines. Some yogurt is high in calcium and some bacterial cultures produce lactase that can help with digestion of lactose. Calcium supplements are also available. Remember, though, that while some foods are high in calcium, the body is unable to use that calcium because other compounds such as oxalates interfere with its absorption. These include foods like Swiss chard, spinach, and rhubarb. Also, calcium can only be absorbed when the body has enough vitamin D, which we get from eggs, liver, and exposure to sunlight. A dietitian can help your family plan meals around lactose intolerance. Before taking such matters into their own hands, parents should keep in mind that taking vitamins and minerals of the wrong kind or in the wrong amounts can be harmful.

If you are lactose intolerant and feel bad, don't. You are in the majority. Most people in the world—and we are speaking globally here—are or become lactose intolerant.

CHAPTER 11

Diarrhea and How to Treat It

FREQUENT LOOSE OR WATERY STOOLS . . . SUNKEN

EYES, DRY MOUTH, DECREASED URINATION . . .

FEVER . . . VOMITING . . . NAUSEA . . .

POOR WEIGHT GAIN, SKINNY MUSCLES . . .

BLOOD IN STOOLS

Across the world, diarrhea represents one of the major health dangers to children. It is the earth's number-one cause of infant mortality, and when it affects a child repeatedly, it leaves him unable to grow normally.

In developing countries, the impact of diarrhea has been improved significantly thanks to better water supplies and hygienic conditions, but still, it remains an extremely common problem—even in the United States. During the winter months particularly, intestinal flu results in many visits to pediatric emergency rooms around the country and an increased number of hospitalizations to manage accompanying severe diarrhea and dehydration.

As a public health issue, diarrhea is not a topic we can deal with casually, but rather one that every parent should learn about in order to minimize its negative impact. If nothing else, the parent provides the first line of defense against dangerous dehydration. But your awareness and understanding of what is happening will not only help prevent dehydration but alert you to when medical attention is needed as well.

What Is Diarrhea?

Like constipation, diarrhea is a relative term. Because all adults and children establish their own individual patterns for frequency of bathroom use and stool consistency, diarrhea is defined as a change in a person's number of stools per day or a change in stool fluidity. For children who regularly have two or three semisoft stools per day, an increase to five stools, even if they are still semisoft, may be called diarrhea. For children who regularly have one stool a day, an increase to three or more might represent diarrhea.

Diarrhea can be divided into three categories: acute diarrhea, chronic diarrhea, and nonspecific diarrhea of childhood. We classify diarrhea as either acute or chronic according to how long it lasts. Acute diarrhea lasts for less than two weeks and is usually caused by food intolerance, a virus, or bacterial or parasitic infection. Chronic diarrhea lasts longer than two weeks and can be caused by conditions such as celiac disease or inflammatory bowel disease, or functional disorders like irritable bowel syndrome. Some parasite infections can also cause chronic diarrhea.

In this chapter, we will discuss both acute and chronic diarrhea, their causes, and usual treatments. Nonspecific diarrhea of childhood, an important cause of chronic diarrhea in toddlers, will be addressed separately in chapter 12. Suffice it to say at this point that nonspecific diarrhea of childhood is a benign form of diarrhea caused by an inability of the digestive tract to handle excessive fluid and can readily be controlled if parents recognize it early.

Acute Diarrhea

Diarrhea is caused, essentially, by inadequate water absorption by the intestine. Normally, the flow of water into and out of the gut is perfectly maintained at appropriate levels. Inflammation, whether from a virus, protein allergy, or other irritant, can throw that balance off. What a parent notices are changes in the stool's fluidity, consistency, and regularity.

How does this happen? Inflammation can affect absorption in two ways: it can decrease the amount of water absorbed and decrease the amount of time that the small and large intestine have to absorb that water. In both cases, larger volumes of fluid reach the colon, and when the colon's ability to reabsorb this fluid is overwhelmed, diarrhea results.

Here's an example that might give a better sense of how closely the intestine fine-tunes its water balance. A healthy fifteen-pound infant will pass about one ounce of stool a day after processing close to one quart of fluid in the colon. If the amount of stool were to increase by just two additional ounces, the stool would be watery and you would immediately know that your baby has developed diarrhea.

COMMON CULPRITS

Gastroenteritis, an inflammation of the intestine most frequently caused by viruses but also by bacteria and parasites, accounts for most cases of acute diarrhea. Also known as intestinal flu, viral gastroenteritis has an incubation period of three to four days, and it's often accompanied by vomiting and mild fever. The impact of gastroenteritis is always potentially more serious in young children than older ones, mainly because the fluid balance is more unstable in the younger child: it takes comparatively less water loss to bring on dehydration.

The list of agents that can cause diarrhea is long and can be divided into three broad groups: viruses, bacteria, and parasites. The following list describes the most common along with their general symptoms to help you identify the offender in particular cases.

MOST COMMON CULPRITS IN ACUTE DIARRHEA	
VIRUSES	CHARACTERISTICS
Adenovirus	Mild diarrhea, vomiting, and fever.
Norwalk agent	Fever, headache, muscle aches lasting for twelve to twenty-four hours. May cause illness in any age group, at any time of the year. Commonly spread by contaminated water or shellfish; often seen at school camps and on cruise ships.
Rotavirus	Affects mostly young children, usually in winter; infants at risk of dehydration. Mild fever is common.
BACTERIA	CHARACTERISTICS
Campylobacter	Often in undercooked foods, such as chicken, causes food poisoning. Thorough cooking will kill this bacteria (180°F for chicken).
Clostridium difficile	A major cause of diarrhea experienced after

continued on next page

BACTERIA	CHARACTERISTICS
	taking antibiotics, *C. difficile* manufactures powerful toxins that cause ulcerations, inflammation, and severe diarrhea that is often bloody and mucusy.
Cholera	Causes severe watery diarrhea and dehydration; cholera outbreaks still occur in parts of Latin America, Asia, and Africa.
Escherichia coli	Contracted mostly from uncooked meats such as hamburger as well as from drinking fresh, unpasteurized apple cider. One strain, *E. coli* 0157:H7, is associated with hemolytic uremic syndrome (HUS), a serious condition that can result in kidney damage.
Salmonella	An important cause of food poisoning, salmonella can present with bloody diarrhea, fever, and nausea. Some individuals "carry" the bacteria in their gastrointestinal tracts without being sick themselves, and can transmit it to others.
Shigella	A particularly virulent bacterium that can cause bloody diarrhea, high fevers, shaking chills, and even seizures.

PARASITES	CHARACTERISTICS
Cryptosporidium	Especially dangerous for people with immunodeficiency issues, such as cancer patients, transplant recipients, and people with HIV or AIDS. Causes a large-volume watery diarrhea and is difficult to cure.
Entamoeba histolytica	The only amoeba that infects the human intestine, *E. histolytica* is transmitted through contaminated water and food and can cause severe ulcers of the intestine with bleeding and fevers. It can also travel through the blood to the liver and form abscesses.

continued on next page

PARASITES	CHARACTERISTICS
Giardia lamblia	One of the most common parasites contracted by children in day-care centers. Heavy infestation with *Giardia* causes malabsorption of fat by the intestine. Many children are "healthy carriers" who show no signs of infection but can infect other playmates around them. Effective treatment is available with antibiotics such as metronidazole or quinacrine.
Pinworms *(Enterobius vermicularis)*	This is the most common parasite in the United States and affects mainly young children. Though it usually lives in the gut, the female parasite crawls out of the anus to lay her eggs, causing intense itching and poor sleep. It is quite contagious. Effective treatment is available and might need to be administered to the whole family or classroom, if the parasite keeps recurring.

SYMPTOMS: WHEN TO WORRY

Diarrhea is usually accompanied by any or all of these symptoms: cramping abdominal pain, bloating, nausea, and an urgent need to use the bathroom. Depending on the cause, fever or bloody stools might also be present. The appearance and smell of the stool often provides, in addition to water, a hint of what is being malabsorbed: when carbohydrates are not being digested and are fermented by the bacteria in the colon, for example, the stools smell of vinegar. (In infants, stool can sometimes be seen foaming in the diaper as a result of the bubbles formed during fermentation. The combination of gas and cramps can cause the stools to be expelled explosively!) If fat is poorly absorbed, stool will be bulky, pale, and shiny.

Sometimes, parents of infants will be unaware of the extent and severity of their baby's diarrhea because water in the stool is promptly absorbed by the diaper. We have seen many children in the emergency room quite dehydrated with parents who thought that despite having little stool they were still urinating well, when in reality the child was not urinating at all (a sign of dehydration) and the wet diaper was all stool water!

SIGNS OF DEHYDRATION

Signs of dehydration in children include not only dry mouth and tongue, a lack of tears, and no wet diapers for three hours or more, but also sunken abdomen, eyes, or cheeks, high fever, listlessness or irritability, and skin that does not flatten when pinched and released. Parents who suspect their child is dehydrated should call their doctor immediately.

THREE LEVELS OF DEHYDRATION	
SEVERITY	SYMPTOMS
Mild	Elevated pulse, dry mouth, no tears
Moderate	Sunken eyes, loose skin, no urine; about 10 percent of body weight lost
Severe	Fifteen percent of body weight lost; state of shock brought on by too little fluid in the arteries and veins

Although the effects of dehydration all sound pretty scary, you should not panic. In the majority of cases, mild and moderate dehydration can be managed quickly with oral hydration fluids, such as Pedialyte, Ricelyte, Infalyte, and others. Only severe dehydration is a life-threatening emergency. Remember: The younger the child, the quicker she can become dehydrated. Be aware that even a few very watery stools in an infant can cause a significant shift in the body's fluid and electrolyte (salt) balance, which can impact the child's health.

PARENT ACTION PLAN

So, what's the first thing a parent should do when diarrhea strikes? Talk to your health care provider. To estimate the severity of the diarrhea, we ask parents questions that help us determine whether the fluid losses are greater than what the child is able to drink and keep in. This is pretty straightforward: if the balance is negative, the risk of dehydration is present and real. Here are some questions to help you determine the urgency of the situation:

- Can your child drink and keep down what he drinks?
- Is he nauseated? Is he vomiting?
- Is there a high fever? (Fever increases the body's fluid requirements, as fluid evaporates when we sweat.)
- Is the stool bloody? (Bloody diarrhea is usually caused by bacterial infections, which might need treatment with antibiotics.)

Treatment

The most effective treatment for acute diarrhea is to maintain hydration with an over-the-counter preparation such as

Pedialyte or Infalyte. Even some sports drinks like Gatorade may be used, though some parents might be uncomfortable with the sugar in them. Other liquids can be used, but they are less effective because they don't contain the right amounts of electrolytes, or body salts such as sodium and potassium. Diarrhea can drain the body of these essential substances, so rehydration must include the replacement of sodium and potassium. In addition a small amount of sugar is necessary because it helps the body absorb the needed salts.

Not all fluid will treat diarrhea effectively. Many commonly used drinks have too much sugar to be safely used: apple juice, for example, has about five times the concentration of sugar of Pedialyte. Such high-sugar drinks pull fluid into the intestine, which is the reverse of what you want to be doing.

GOOD AND NOT GOOD: LIQUIDS FOR REHYDRATION	
GOOD	
Pedialyte/Infalyte, or similar proprietary product	Best choice, as they include electrolytes and a little sugar.
Sports drinks, such as Gatorade	Generally good choice; include some electrolytes and sugar.
Water	Okay to use, but electrolytes need to be provided, too—otherwise, hyponatremia (low sodium in the blood) can develop.
NOT GOOD	
Soda	Too much sugar in most sodas, and no salt: counterproductive.

continued on next page

NOT GOOD	
Tea	No electrolytes; risk of hyponatremia.
Fruit juices*	Most have too much sugar and insufficient electrolytes: counterproductive. Prune, apple, and pear juices should particularly be avoided, as they contain sorbitol, which promotes diarrhea, gas, and cramps

*See chapter 12 on nonspecific diarrhea of childhood and juice abuse.

ANTIBIOTICS: A WORD OF CAUTION

Because most diarrhea is caused by viruses, antibiotics are of little use in its treatment. This is an important point, because parents often feel antibiotics are helpful for all types of infection. Giving antibiotics to your child when she has a viral infection, however, is not only ineffective, but it can change for the worse the balance of good bacteria that live in the gut. Remember that antibiotics destroy many bacteria that *belong* in our large intestines—ones that help stave off infection by disease-producing bacteria, and others whose very presence prevents overgrowth of toxin-producing bacteria like *C. difficile*. In fact, it has been found that patients—kids and grownups alike—taking antibiotics for the treatment of salmonella are more likely to become carriers of that bacterium than those who leave it to their immune system to battle, which means that even when they might not be sick anymore, they harbor the bacteria in their intestines and can pass it on to those with whom they come in contact. It is better to let the body fight viral gastroenteritis infection without interference from antibiotics whenever possible. Diarrhea will stop when the body's immune system produces antibodies against the virus. The body will usually free itself of the invading virus in a week or two at most.

There are exceptions to this guideline. A baby who is less than three months old and infected with salmonella or shigella *has* to be treated with antibiotics. The protective barrier in the intestine of the very young child is less effective than in the older child, and bacteria can escape the intestine and get into the bloodstream, where it can cause a more serious infection. An immunocompromised child is similarly vulnerable, and may require antibiotics as well.

The situation may also be different for someone whose immune system isn't functioning well. In such cases, simple viral diarrhea can last for months and possibly cause more severe and long-lasting damage to the intestinal lining. Immunodeficiency might be the product of medication being taken for another condition or a problem in manufacturing the disease-fighting proteins called immunoglobulins (or, as one patient put it in a tribute to Pac-Man, "immunogobblings"!). When the immune system is compromised, patients should follow their practitioner's regimen.

PROTECTIVE-BUBBLE CAUTION

Before you think of keeping your child in a protective bubble in an effort to avoid any possibility of exposure to infection, consider this: it is believed that a lack of exposure to bacteria early in life might be an important factor in the increased incidence of

**chronic inflammatory bowel and respiratory diseases
in children over the past few decades.**

**In a 2002 Swiss study, children living near farms
and thereby exposed to all kinds of molds and pollen
showed fewer allergic diseases than city children who
had fewer natural allergens in their environment.
Too much sterility in our environment and food
supply might not be good for us and, in fact, might
prevent the immune system from developing
appropriate responses to infectious organisms. The
immune system may attack itself rather than a
bacteria or a parasite, for example, because it can't
recognize the intruder.**

TRAVELER'S DIARRHEA

Traveler's diarrhea is an infectious acute diarrhea often contracted when traveling to places with poor sanitation, substandard, food preparation, and/or contaminated water. It is more prevalent in such areas as Latin America, Africa, Asia, and the Middle East than in the United States, Canada, or Europe. The most common culprits are strains of *E. coli* and parasites.

This diarrhea can be accompanied by severe cramping and fever, muscle aches, and vomiting. If bleeding accompanies the diarrhea, antibiotics such as ciprofloxacin or a sulfa drug are routinely prescribed. The following precautions can be taken to help prevent traveler's diarrhea:

- Do not drink tap water or use it to brush your teeth
- Do not use ice made from tap water

- Do not drink unpasteurized milk or dairy products
- Avoid all raw fruits and vegetables you haven't peeled yourself
- Do not eat raw or rare meat and fish
- Do not eat meat or shellfish that is not hot when served to you
- Do not eat food from street vendors

Bottled water and carbonated soft drinks are safe, provided you can open the bottle yourself.

Chronic Diarrhea

As described so far, the main impact of most diarrheas is on the balance of fluid and salts in the body. Acute diarrhea, however, can deteriorate into a more long-lasting, or chronic, disturbance as a result of the damage to the intestines done by the virus, parasite, or bacteria causing the diarrhea.

When does acute diarrhea turn chronic? A diarrhea that lasts over two weeks is categorized as chronic. Sometimes, when the bowel movements alternate between well-formed and not-so-normal ones, parents often have a hard time remembering exactly when their child's diarrhea actually started. The following questions will help to recall onset as accurately as possible and in many cases provide important clues to help us identify possible causes:

- Was there an initial viral infection or any fever, congestion, cough, rash, or similar condition?
- Did she receive an antibiotic?
- Were other (nonantibiotic) medications that could possibly cause damage to the intestine prescribed?
- Was a new food introduced recently?

- Are there associated symptoms such as a cough? A rash? Joint swelling?
- Are any other family members similarly affected?
- Has he had similar episodes before?

CAUSES

Chronic diarrhea results from conditions that interfere with the absorption of nutrients in the small intestine, or from disturbed fluid reabsorption of water in the large intestine. Because digestion and absorption of food are complicated and require many steps, the list of potential culprits is long and includes, but is not confined to, food allergies or intolerance (to sorbitol or fructose, for example), celiac disease, inflammatory bowel disease, cystic fibrosis, and medications.

When searching for the cause of diarrhea, it also helps to remember what is involved in digesting food normally (see chapter 1 for a more detailed explanation) and what happens when any of the steps fail. For example, the villi (those minute projections covering the intestinal wall) may be damaged by anything from severe infections by viruses or parasites to reactions to protein allergies or wheat-containing products.

DIAGNOSIS

When a child develops chronic diarrhea and experiences poor weight gain, referral to a pediatric gastroenterologist will help get to the bottom of the problem without undue delays. The causes are not always obvious, and there are many possibilities to explore. The first question, of course, is whether the child is actually eating enough. This might seem self-evident, but often we need food diaries and precise accounts of everything offered to the child to eat before we can rule out the possibility that a particular or limited diet is responsible for the diarrhea and weight loss. In a food diary, we ask parents and caregivers to choose three to five representative days and list, in as much detail as possible, everything the child eats and drinks, recording ounces, portion sizes (spices, tablespoons, and so forth), and brand names; the time of day when the meals are eaten; the times of any bowel movements, and descriptions of the bowel movements.

With this information and using available food databases, we can calculate the proportions of fat, protein, and carbohydrates in the child's typical diet. We can also begin to focus on specific components of the diet, such as items containing cow's-milk protein, certain carbohydrates, or fats, as causes of the problem. From that point, diet can be modified or tests conducted to explore other potential reasons for malabsorption and diarrhea. Intestinal biopsies obtained by endoscopy, for example, will let us know if celiac disease is the culprit, while cystic fibrosis can be identified through a sweat test.

MANAGEMENT

The three keys to managing chronic diarrhea are identifying the cause, providing appropriate treatment, and reversing the malnutrition caused by the condition. Treatment might include initial rehydration and changes in the diet to exclude certain foods. Special formulas and supplements are often prescribed as well. The wide array of specialized foods available today is of great help and frequently prevents the need for hospitalization or complex intravenous feedings. Reversing the malnutrition is critical in helping the child recover and lead a normal life, and this part of the process requires intensive investigation and follow-up. Teamwork with a dietitian or nutritionist makes the task more manageable.

POST-GASTROENTERITIS SYNDROME

Another important cause of chronic diarrhea is the so-called post-gastroenteritis syndrome. Typically, the child first appears to have had a run-of-the-mill intestinal flu, only to continue having loose stools and not seem to be able to fully recover. Weight loss becomes apparent after a few weeks, and every effort to clear the diarrhea with formula or diet changes fails. The child's nutritional condition spirals down and physical examination raises lots of concerns about thinness and muscle wasting.

In a young infant or child, the effects of this ongoing food intolerance and malabsorption can be devastating. Small children have few energy reserves, but their calorie and protein requirements are very high, so any disruptions will result in a serious failure to thrive. A vicious cycle develops: the damaged intestine and poor absorption cause progressive malnutrition, and, in turn, the malnutrition prevents the lining from healing. The normal function of enzymes, pancreas, and liver, as well as all body functions in charge of recovery, are thrown out of balance.

Luckily, we are now able to provide children afflicted by this serious condition with sufficient intravenous nutrition during the long periods needed for complete healing of the intestine. This intravenous nutrition delivers concentrated mixtures of protein, sugar, and fat through special catheters placed in large veins. This technique is known by its initials, TPN, for total parenteral nutrition. ("Parenteral" refers to the administration through a vein as opposed to *enteral*, which means through the intestine.) It's not an exaggeration to say that this technology has changed the course of medicine and has allowed us to save many lives that might otherwise have been lost to malnutrition.

IMMUNODEFICIENCY

A final cause of chronic diarrhea that must be addressed is immunodeficiency, or defects in natural defenses. Some are congenital, while others, like HIV/AIDS, are acquired. Often, a deficiency will be identified when the baby is three to four months old when the immunity inherited from the mother's circulation diminishes and the baby's own immune system begins, or should begin, kicking in. A child with immunodeficiency will not be able to effectively make this transition and will be at risk for infections that the body usually eliminates.

Diarrhea is a common problem in children, one that parents need to be aware of and understand. Maintaining hydration and nutrition are two of the crucial functions of the intestine. When this capacity is affected by viruses, bacteria, or parasites, or when the intestinal lining is damaged, serious consequences often follow, for which diarrhea might be just the outward sign. You can help minimize the impact of these infections by understanding how to prevent dehydration and maintain the nutrition of your child. Parents must know when a change in stool frequency and consistency requires medical help.

CHAPTER 12

Nonspecific Diarrhea of Childhood

Nonspecific diarrhea of childhood, often called toddler's diarrhea because of the age group it most commonly affects, needs to be recognized for what it is: a benign condition that tends to improve, sometimes dramatically, with simple changes in diet or by the time a child is about three years old. It is a puzzling and frustrating type of diarrhea, however, because it occurs in otherwise healthy toddlers who, no matter how many times they are examined by a pediatrician and how many attempts at removing dairy products—for suspected lactose intolerance or milk allergy—from the diet, continue to pass frequent and often very large bowel movements.

The truth is, children with nonspecific diarrhea are not actually sick! They have loose stools, but no major symptoms other than possibly some extra gas and cramps before a bowel movement. The volume of diarrhea is high, of course—from five to ten stools per day—but the foods that parents are able to identify in the diapers (undigested peas or carrots, for example), about which they worry so much, are simply fiber-containing foods that none of us can efficiently digest. You should know that the presence of these foods, and the diarrhea in general, is not a reflection of poor digestion or an enzyme deficiency. Steady growth, as tracked by your health care provider, is the best proof that this diarrhea is not affecting your child's health.

As in all cases of diarrhea, the health care provider will explore the possibility of food intolerance, parasite infection, drug side effects, or underlying conditions like celiac disease. If those can all be ruled out, a diagnosis of toddler's diarrhea can be made with confidence.

Juice Abuse

One of the biggest culprits in nonspecific diarrhea is excessive juice consumption. Parents are usually taken by surprise when we discuss "juice abuse" as the reason for their child's diarrhea. How can juice be abused? Isn't it an excellent source of vitamin C? And, furthermore, isn't juice a smart way to keep a child well hydrated if she's losing liquid through her watery stools?

As we discussed in chapter 11, the sugar in juice actually pulls extra water into the intestine, and the natural acids in juice stimulate contractions, thereby speeding the transit of the water, and material accompanying it, through the gut. This deprives the surface of the intestine of the time it needs to do the job of absorbing fluid and nutrients.

Juice is basically lots of sugar in liquid form. An eight-ounce juice box, for example, usually contains about 26 grams of sugar, the equivalent of 120 calories. In contrast, an orange or half an apple will provide a child with just as much vitamin C, but with only half the calories. Moreover, excessive juice consumption is now recognized as a reason for poor weight gain in some children and obesity in others, for in addition to providing lots of empty (nonnutritive) calories, juices suppress an appetite for "real" food. And children drinking excessive amounts of juice are also commonly found to be calcium-deficient, and eat little protein-rich foods.

There's no doubt that some children will get hooked on juice and will resist any encouragement to drink water as long as they still believe that there's juice available, like when they still see it sitting on the refrigerator shelf. Using juice sparingly so as to avoid forming a habit in the first place is the best advice, but if it's too late for preventive measures, parents should know that it's worth the struggle to wean a child off juice and back to water as a thirst-quencher.

Consequences of Juice Abuse

Even in the absence of diarrhea, the consequences of excessive juice intake can be serious. A juice-filled bottle used as a pacifier, for example, will expose a child's teeth to the damaging effects of fermented sugars and acids. Most parents have usually heard of milk rot, or bottle-baby syndrome, in infants, the terrible damage to the enamel that takes place as a result of sleeping with the bottle in the mouth. Mouth bacteria will work just as happily on the sugar in juice as they will on the sugar in milk, and the end result is a literal eating away of the teeth. In summary, juice abuse can cause or exacerbate diarrhea and counteract attempts at rehydration, and promote tooth decay in bottle-fed babies. It can also decrease fat and protein intake and, in some cases, promote obesity.

By avoiding juice abuse, parents will go a long way toward preventing nonspecific diarrhea of childhood and a host of other problems. Parents can easily recognize this kind of diarrhea and work, if not to prevent it, to control it and ultimately reverse it. The measures are simple and the long-term benefits can be substantial.

The Important Role of Dietary Fat

In the past few years, we've learned that fat has important effects on the way the intestine moves food along. First of all, it slows down the rate at which food is emptied from the stomach, so nutrients are delivered to the small intestine slowly enough so that they can be well absorbed. Fat also slows down intestinal contractions and hence lengthens food's transit through the small intestine. The effect of fat is therefore welcome to anyone for whom rapid passage of food and liquids through the intestine is an issue. If added to the diet of a child with toddler's diarrhea, fat will help to improve the situation greatly.

As already discussed in chapter 2, fat is an important component of a balanced diet, and should provide an average of 30 percent of the calories the child consumes daily. Not only does it help intestinal function, but the growing brain needs essential fatty acids and cholesterol as well as fat-soluble vitamins. Because fat plays such an important role in the young child's development, we do not recommend low-fat milk until after a child has turned three years old.

Treatment

Treatment for nonspecific diarrhea is aimed at reducing the load of fluid that the intestine needs to work on as well as slowing down that fluid's transit through the intestine. It is not difficult to come up with a few practical recommendations; some children will have a firm stool within days of instituting the following three simple steps:

- Take juice away *completely*
- In toddlers decrease daily fluid intake to no more than fourteen to twenty ounces, all of it given in the form of whole milk or water
- Increase the amount of fat in the diet

Parents and relatives are often surprised to hear a nutrition expert recommending a high-fat diet: "Are you really telling me not to worry about his cholesterol?" they ask. "You mean fried chicken and french fries, cheese omelets, and fish sticks?" The answer is yes. The addition of fat will bring a needed balance to what was probably a sugar-rich diet. Try it! Of course, once the diarrhea is resolved, make sure that the diet goes back to a more balanced one. (See chapter 2 and the recommendations of the New Food Pyramid.)

CHAPTER 13

Constipation and Withholding

SWOLLEN STOMACH . . .

DIMINISHED APPETITE . . . BLOOD IN STOOL . . .

SOILING OF UNDERPANTS

Constipation is a very common problem: probably one of every four patients seen by a gastroenterologist is there for stooling difficulties. In a general practitioner's office, constipation is an everyday complaint.

In this chapter, we will define childhood constipation and provide suggestions to help identify it in a timely manner so that unnecessary discomfort can be avoided. It is important that constipation be addressed appropriately and promptly, as it can lead to stool withholding in some children. Withholding is the leading cause of soiling, or *encopresis*, the embarrassing but involuntary passage of a bowel movement in the underpants. This can be one of the most frustrating complications of constipation that the specialist is asked to resolve.

What Is Functional Constipation?

Functional constipation may be defined as the passage of two stools or fewer per week for at least twelve consecutive weeks. Stools that are passed are large in diameter, and accompanying symptoms may include fecal soiling, irritability, abdominal cramps, and diminished appetite—all of which tend to disappear immediately with the passage of a large stool. A very important component of the definition is the level of discomfort associated with passing stool. Frequency, in fact, is not as important as what the stool is like and what the child experiences as she passes it.

What Causes Constipation?

Constipation is the result of four major factors that influence the child's ability to pass stool normally: dietary factors that affect how much water is present in the bowel movement, the effectiveness of the muscle contractions responsible for propelling the stool along the intestine, the voluntary control of the anal sphincter at the time of toilet training, and, finally, the integrity of the nerves and muscles participating in the expulsion of the stool.

The Role of Diet

The role played by diet in constipation has to be clarified. For example, many people think that milk, cheese, or chocolate *causes* constipation, but the problem is not inherent in these foods. The basic fact is that when children eat such items in generous amounts, they simultaneously cut back on their intake of fruits, vegetables, and other high-fiber foods. It is the lack of roughage that causes constipation, not the milk or chocolate.

When a child is constipated, stool builds up and overfills the large intestine. The consequent overstretching causes a diffuse pain below the belly button, and the child will frequently grab the lower belly or even point right above the pelvis. When stools are wide and hurt on the way out the rectum, the child will indicate the buttocks as the source of his discomfort ("My tushy hurts").

Constipation can also be associated with a general lack of appetite and with mood changes. Typically, a constipated child will be clingy or cranky, and she will start eating, only to stop in the middle of the meal and appear unhappy. The stool buildup causes increased pain every time food is taken in, because of the gastrocolic reflex. But this is not a result of being totally backed up: the stool is only accumulating in the large intestine, and it is nowhere close to the stomach!

Treatment

Prevention is one of the best treatments for constipation. The key is to increase the fiber in the diet and ensure adequate fluid intake: these two steps will help to avert pain when the stool moves along the colon. An effective routine to avoid constipation involves attention to the following areas:

☺ Sufficient fluid intake
☺ Sufficient fiber intake

☺ Regular exercise

☺ Anticipatory guidance to prevent stool withholding

In some children, increasing fiber intake can be quite difficult because they simply are incapable of eating enough fruits, vegetables, and wholesome cereals to make a difference. In such cases, a variety of fiber supplements (such as Benefiber, Metamucil, or Konsyl), fiber-enriched juices, or prune juice and dried fruits (which contain natural stimulants) could be used.

When a diet cannot be modified sufficiently to prevent overdrying of the stools, various stool softeners are available. Gastroenterologists prescribe them routinely so that kids don't have to suffer through painful bowel movements. Some of the most commonly used softeners include MiraLax, Colace, mineral oil, and Kondremul (a mix of mineral oil and fiber): all are effective and nonhabit forming. Stimulant laxatives, such as Senokot, on the other hand, tend to cause cramping and should be avoided for long-term use.

THE NUMBERS TELL THE STORY

The National Institutes of Health (NIH) report that constipation is the most common gastrointestinal complaint in the United States, responsible for about two million doctor visits annually. However, most adults treat themselves without seeking medical help, as is evident from the $725 million Americans spend on laxatives each year!

Anal Malformations

Before the diet is changed and stool softeners are used, the presence of an anorectal malformation should be ruled out. In these conditions, the anus might be too small or covered with a membrane, or even situated too far forward. A simple visual examination and rectal exam can be of great benefit, because missing the diagnosis for years might result in misplaced efforts to control abnormal stooling without ever resolving the problem. In some instances of anorectal malformations, surgical intervention may be needed.

In children with the congenital spinal defect spina bifida or a tethered spinal cord, the anal sphincter reflexes will be abnormal and may cause constipation. A neurological examination complemented by a CT scan or MRI will determine the diagnosis and guide appropriate treatment.

Infant Straining (Dyschezia)

"Dyschezia" is a word used to describe infantile difficulty in passing a bowel movement. The infant will strain, turn red, draw up his legs, and appear to be in obvious discomfort until a soft, sometimes even loose, stool is passed. The condition is caused by a discoordination of the muscles involved in stool expulsion: in order to pass the stool, the rectal muscles have to relax at the same time that the abdominal wall muscles contract. If the sphincter is contracting while the baby is pushing, she's going to turn red and no stool will come out.

Dyschezia is a functional problem caused by immaturity and will resolve itself in a matter of a few weeks or months as the baby matures and her muscles learn to work in synchronicity.

MANAGING CONSTIPATION	
INTERVENTION	PRACTICAL SUGGESTIONS
Clear the compacted stools filling the rectum	Oral laxatives similar to the ones used before undergoing a colonoscopy can be used, such as MiraLax. This preparation contains polyethylene glycol (PEG) and is not habit forming. Enemas should be avoided as much as possible, but if there is a large fecal mass, an enema might be the most direct and effective way to begin successful long-term management. If parents are insecure or too anxious, this procedure can be done in the doctor's office.
Eliminate all possible sources of rectal pain and discomfort	Avoid use of irritating wipes. Treat rashes and skin abrasions. Use emolients such as A&D ointment, Aquaphor, or Desitin.
Provide a laxative regimen for maintenance	Use a nonhabit-forming laxative. Use effective toileting routines (behavior modification—allows the muscle structures to go back to normal size and to function properly).
Institute new routines for bathroom use	Sitting at the toilet at certain times of the day, best after meals. Positive reinforcement after successful bowel movements.

What Is Stool Withholding?

Stool withholding, or functional fecal retention, is the most common cause of constipation and soiling in children. It is defined by repetitive attempts to avoid passing stool because of fear of pain associated with moving the bowels. The child learns to contract the muscles of the pelvis in response to the urge, and a large amount of stool progressively accumulates in the rectum. All of the child's behaviors and symptoms (stiffening, holding on to furniture, turning red, crying) are explained by the voluntary effort to avoid pain.

In some cases, there might be no normal movement for two, four, or even eight weeks, but at some point, incontinence finally occurs. When the muscles get tired and relax, the child will have an accident, soiling the underpants. This can happen when the child is asleep or when passing gas.

When I saw Fran in the office, she was a vivacious and precocious four-year-old who had no problems toilet training. Recently, though, the parents had started to note a peculiar and puzzling behavior: Fran would run to a quiet corner of the house and seem to focus intently while assuming an oddly stiff and funny posture. She twirled back and forth while uttering small grunts, turned red, and sometimes even broke out in a sweat. This would pass within a few minutes, and she went right back to play. Meanwhile, Fran was skipping one or two days between her bowel movements, and when she finally went, they were wider than normal and she was clearly in pain. It took some convincing to make Fran's parents understand that what appeared to be straining to pass a movement was actually active withholding to *not* let it out!

WHY DOES IT HAPPEN?

The anus is an area very rich with nerve fibers. They are needed to help us sense the difference between liquid and solid stool, and also to accurately detect the presence of gas. Because there are so many nerve endings, any small cut, irritation, or rash in the rectal area will be very painful.

In stool withholding, the child is trying to avoid pain by squeezing the rectal muscles and pushing the stool back, away from the sensitive area. As a result, the feeling of urgency subsides, and days or weeks can be skipped between passing stools. But this relief comes at a price: as they are held, stools become larger, drier, and progressively more painful to evacuate. A vicious cycle sets in.

In the older child, "doody dancing" develops, as the child contorts and postures to avoid passing a stool. Turning red, sweating, and stiffening while holding on to the furniture or to the parents are all variations of this reaction. Many parents misinterpret what the child is trying to do, but the dance, and withholding, should be a clear signal that something needs to be done to prevent the problem from spiraling out of control.

TREATMENT

Initial treatment for stool withholding is to relieve the impaction caused by the accumulated stools. In most cases, the specialist will eschew enemas and rely instead on cleansing solutions such as MiraLax, Golytely, or Nulytely. Once the impaction is cleared, parents should concentrate on maintaining habits that will keep stools soft such as encouraging regular intake of fiber and sufficient fluids, establishing consistent toilet routines, and avoiding anything that might cause irritation around the anus.

Reconditioning your child to have regular movements can take time and patience, for the tendency to withhold and the fear of letting go does not disappear immediately. Positive conditioning—like that used in toilet training—can be very successful in retraining.

Involuntary Soiling (Encopresis)

Encopresis is the accidental passing of stools after an age when the child is expected to be toilet trained. Surveys suggest that encopresis might affect up to 1.5 percent of children. It should be anticipated in any child with stubborn constipation, and parents should be prepared to take preventive measures, as it can create a great deal of anxiety, embarrassment, and tension in the family.

Encopresis is usually caused by chronic constipation. When stool is withheld, the rectum is progressively overstretched until the child loses the ability to sense the presence of stool. When the message is consistently disregarded, the brain eventually grows to accept the distension as the normal state, and ignores the signals.

Eventually, when gas is passed—and it needs to be passed regularly—the stool at the rectum will seep through, resulting in soiling. At this point, the child has, for all practical purposes, lost control over his anal sphincter. Parents can't understand how he can be totally unaware that stool is coming out, not to mention be oblivious to the revolting smell of feces emanating from his underpants. One explanation is that children with encopresis often develop a coping mechanism based on denial. The sad part is that they really are, in great measure, adapted to this new situation and are not lying when they claim the seepage "just happens."

It is an exasperating situation, with parents often believing their child is soiling on purpose. Parents' reactions are contradictory, swinging from patient and sympathetic to angry and demanding. The stress in the household mounts with differences of opinion on how to approach the child: bribe or punish? Demand or ignore? Have her wash her own underpants? Just keep on buying new ones? The best approach is to understand the underlying reasons for the soiling and to institute a consistent plan of action while maintaining an emotionally even attitude toward the accidents.

TREATMENT

It goes without saying that the best treatment for encopresis is to avoid stool withholding by managing constipation effectively at the earliest possible time. Two important preventive measures any parent can take are to: (1) recognize that pain accompanying passing stool can result in withholding; and (2) anticipate the developmental stage around eighteen to twenty-four months of age during which successful toilet training occurs. The early warning signs of withholding caused by local irritation or by the development of painful movements should not be ignored.

When a child with encopresis is brought to the specialist for consultation, parents feel great relief when they find out that the soiling is not due to a serious neurological problem affecting their child's capacity to pass a stool normally. It is also comforting for them to hear that the problem has a solution, and that their child will regain continence—and confidence—in time.

Other Causes of Fecal Soiling

Some children experience soiling unrelated to packing of the rectum with stool. Reasons can be physical or psychological. In some cases, the problem is abnormal sensation in the rectal area resulting from inflammation, as seen with infections, or a lack of awareness of rectal function, which is most often seen in children with developmental disorders like autism or mental retardation. In the former case, the inflammation should be evaluated and treated if possible, while in the latter case behavior modification can often be quite effective. Another factor may be abnormal family dynamics, with the soiling being a psychiatric manifestation of anger or stress. *Nonretentive fecal soiling,* as this condition is termed, is more difficult to manage. Psychiatric care is usually recommended and may in fact be necessary to help resolve the conflicts being expressed.

HIRSCHSPRUNG'S DISEASE

Finally, we need to mention Hirschsprung's disease as a possible cause of constipation, even though most children with this condition are diagnosed during infancy. Nevertheless, we do see older children who are treated for years for severe constipation in whom the possibility of Hirschsprung's is raised. It is therefore a significant condition to understand and keep in mind.

Hirschsprung's disease is caused by a lack of nerve, or ganglion, cells in the colon. These cells usually travel the intestine all the way to the anus, but sometimes fail to reach their final destination so that parts of the intestine have no nerve function. Without the nerve cells, the muscles of the rectum cannot relax and remain in constant spasm. Infants so afflicted will have a distended abdomen and vomit bile, as if they had a blockage.

Most children with Hirschsprung's disease are diagnosed shortly after birth or in the first few months of life. Diagnosis is quickly made with X-ray films and confirmed when the biopsies of the intestine show the absence of nerve cells. At this point, corrective surgery is performed.

A Parting Word of Encouragement . . .

Understanding the mechanics of passing a stool, the developmental stages leading to toilet training, and the presentation of stool withholding will help you avoid some of the problems frequently encountered with these processes. Pain avoidance is a powerful deterrent to letting go of a bowel movement, and children will do whatever they can to avoid the overstretching and pain that result when stool is wide and dry. Adjustments in the diet to include the introduction of more fiber-rich food, consuming plenty of fluids, and, in some cases, the use of stool softeners are effective measures that will promote regularity. Getting over the hurdle of toilet training is a milestone that you as parents are entitled to look forward to.

IV

When It's More Than Just Pain

CHAPTER 14

Choosing a Pediatric Gastroenterologist

Consulting a specialist is not the first step one takes in order to address many of the issues discussed in this book. Your pediatrician or family physician knows a great deal about many of the digestive problems that can affect your child; in fact, most of the common upsets such as diarrhea or uncomplicated constipation, spitting up, and bellyaches are considered "bread-and-butter" pediatrics. A pediatrician will provide effective advice and treatment, with no need to consult a gastroenterologist. Referral to a specialist, whether a neurologist, dermatologist, or pediatric gastroenterologist is only considered when management of the problem in the normal way does not bring about the expected results and the complaint does not get resolved or worsens.

Getting a Referral

Most often, a referral to a gastroenterologist will come directly from your primary care doctor, who is usually an excellent source for referral because the specialist is likely to be someone your pediatrician has worked with in the past, been liked by other patients referred to him, and has successfully managed complicated cases.

Upon referral, the pediatrician usually shares the child's medical history, providing the specialist with important information that can help determine the next steps for your child's care. General practitioners and specialists tend to work together closely, often developing trusting relationships that offer the patient an excellent team approach to tackling an aching tummy or more complex digestive disorders. Referrals can also come from friends or relatives who have experienced similar problems or know others who have.

What Should I Know about My Specialist?

It is useful to know certain information about the specialist you are going to see, such as the training, background, and special interests he or she might have. Here are some specific facts to know about a potential specialist:

- Where patients are admitted for procedures and for diagnostic tests
- GI Board certification
- Special areas of interest in the field of gastrointestinal diseases
- Medical school or teaching-hospital affiliation

If you're lucky, you may even know someone who has also been under the care of that doctor, from whom you can get some sense of his or her practice style.

EDUCATION AND TRAINING

An extensive process of training and qualification has been designed to ensure that those practicing medicine do so according to standards that are set and monitored by various formal institutions. The intention is, of course, to maintain high-quality training. How does this translate for a specialist in children's digestive diseases?

Following residency training in general pediatrics, which usually lasts three years, the pediatrician enters a three-year pediatric gastroenterology fellowship program. Accreditation of these programs is overseen by the Accreditation Council of Graduate Medical Education (ACGME) and is quite involved and lengthy, entailing extensive review and evaluation of curriculum, teaching, and staff qualifications.

During specialty training, the pediatric gastroenterology (or GI, for "gastrointestinal") fellows are exposed to and handle an array of difficult cases, the sort normally referred to teaching hospitals. During these three years, they learn how to manage digestive diseases under the supervision of more experienced physicians. Following many hours of hands-on experience, and after taking the Pediatrics Certification Boards, a fellow will take the Pediatric GI Board certification exam, as established in 1990 and administered by the American Board of Medical Specialties (ABMS). The reward for passing is a designation of "board certified in pediatric gastroenterology": now you know what those five words in a doctor's biography represent!*

---

*A specialist is said to be "board qualified"—as opposed to "board certified"—if all training requirements are completed but the qualifying exam has not yet been passed. Recertification exams are currently required every four years, ensuring that doctors stay up to date in their field.

A Little Chemistry

Once a referral is made, developing a good rapport with your doctor, no matter what the specialty, is a key element in managing the stress that comes with having a sick child. You need to feel comfortable with the doctor at the time of the visit. And, looking to the future, as your child reaches adolescence, his rapport with the doctor will become increasingly important.

While recognizing that specialists are consulted for their knowledge and expertise, information needs to flow in both directions for care to be successful. When patients (or patients' parents) feel at ease, they will probably provide more details when relating their child's history, and it is through these details that crucial information is revealed. If a parent feels inhibited by a style they feel is unsympathetic, or a manner that seems gruff, those details may be left out, making a definitive diagnosis harder to reach.

As a parent, you need to feel that your child is the center of attention during the visit and that your feelings are understood and taken seriously. You can usually tell the difference between someone who is listening closely as you speak and someone who is clearly preoccupied with problems other than your own. If you arrive with certain questions and concerns that need to be addressed, make sure to raise them before the appointment ends. Keep a list and refer to it during your visit: it will keep you focused and provide you with the reassurance that you covered all the important points. Having served as the primary "digestive detective" before meeting with the specialist, you will be in a better position to know whether the points that *you* felt were important were taken into consideration.

In a nutshell: Taking care of a sick child requires teamwork between parents and doctors. The success of your referral to a pediatric gastroenterologist ultimately will be evident when you feel a part of that team and can see an improvement in your child's condition.

CHAPTER 15

Celiac Disease: More Than Bellyaches and Diarrhea

Celiac disease is an immune response caused by intolerance to wheat, rye, and barley. Though the distinction may be confusing, it is not an allergy: in fact, celiac disease is a permanent, immune-mediated abnormal response to specific proteins in those cereals. It is also known as celiac sprue, non-tropical sprue ("sprue" refers to the malabsorption characteristic of the condition), and gluten-sensitive enteropathy (damage to the intestine).

Emily was referred to me by her pediatrician, who was concerned about the horrible smell of Emily's bowel movements. Emily was still formula fed, but over the past nine months since her birth, cereals, and then vegetables—she loved her carrots and sweet potatoes—had been introduced to her diet. She had become slightly constipated on rice, but by the time I saw her, she was already on oatmeal, barley, and mixed cereals. The only thing out of the ordinary was her stool. In addition to the strong smell, the bulk of the stool had increased to the point of overflowing her diapers. Meanwhile, Emily, who had been so even tempered, was now becoming cranky and restless, seemed hungry all day long, and slept poorly. She cried throughout the office visit, even when offered the bottle. Her complexion was pale, her ribs showed, and her belly was like a balloon. With that, the signs and symptoms were all there: Emily's diagnosis of celiac disease was confirmed by endoscopy, and a gluten-free diet has helped her fully recover and become herself again.

At the root of celiac disease is an intolerance to gluten. What is gluten? Gluten is what remains after dough is washed to remove starch and it consists of a mix of proteins. It's what makes dough sticky, and what makes a baker happy: the changes in the proteins of gluten, together with yeast fermentation causes a loaf of bread to feel light, airy, and chewy when you bite into it. In people with celiac disease, gluten triggers an immune-system response.

Celiac disease causes damage to the villi, the slender finger-like projections of the small intestine that are responsible for absorbing food. As a result of this damage, absorption of nutrients is less than complete, and not only nutrients but calories are lost. That's why there is poor weight gain, or even weight loss, in celiac disease patients.

Celiac disease, however, causes more than just localized damage to the intestine. Because it involves the immune system, other parts of the body may be affected, most commonly the skin, thyroid gland, and bones. Celiac patients often develop a very peculiar type of rash called *dermatitis herpetiformis* (because it resembles the blisters caused by herpes-virus infection), making the skin itchy, red, and blistery. This rash will get better when gluten is eliminated from the diet. Dermatologists are familiar with this condition, but general practitioners might not see it often.

Typical vs. Atypical

For years, celiac disease was believed to be rare in the United States. This was always something of a puzzle, given the fact that so many Americans have European ancestors. Sure enough, over the past decade, we have begun to realize that celiac disease is probably just as common this side of the Atlantic as it is in Europe and that the difficulties in diagnosis were mainly because medical professionals were all looking for classical, or "textbook," cases. We were taught in medical school that children with celiac disease developed a malabsorption syndrome after six months of life, following the introduction of solid foods including cereals. They lost weight and were cranky, and their bellies looked very prominent, while their stools were pale, bulky, and very foul smelling.

As it turns out, Emily's classic presentation is not necessarily the typical one anymore; symptomatologies have changed and we now recognize that "atypical" celiac disease might be much more common. This knowledge has come as adult diagnoses of celiac disease have increased: with affected parents often come affected children, and few present as textbook cases. It is clear that those with typical celiac are just the tip of the iceberg.

What prompted these parents to be evaluated for celiac disease in the first place? Iron deficiency anemia, often, and osteoporosis in many other cases. In recent surveys of adults with celiac disease, these two conditions were among the highest on the list of presenting symptoms, though irritable bowel syndrome and other vague intestinal complaints—including constipation and obesity!—are also right up there. Once an adult is diagnosed with celiac disease, their children should undergo screening blood tests to see whether they are at risk of also having the condition.

Heredity

As may be surmised, celiac disease definitely runs in families. The catch is that, contrary to other well-understood genetic disorders like cystic fibrosis or albinism, the risk in children cannot be exactly calculated. In cystic fibrosis, for example, if both parents are carriers, the risk is one in four that one of their children will be born with the disease. In celiac disease, not only is more than one gene involved, but other factors (such as infection or environmental factors) seem to affect the odds as well, so there is currently no way to accurately predict whether a child of a celiac patient will inherit the condition.

It is important nevertheless to identify celiac disease as early as possible, because the longer the intestine is exposed to gluten, and the longer the abnormal immune responses to gluten go on, the chances of developing other immune conditions such as diabetes, thyroid inflammation, or arthritis increase. Long-term exposure of the intestine to gluten damages the tissues repeatedly, increasing the risk for certain intestinal cancers.

How Common Is Celiac Disease?

You might be surprised to learn that celiac disease is the most common genetic condition among Caucasians. The carrier rate in European surveys is about 1 in 200 to 300 people, and when blood screens for celiac disease were performed on a large number of volunteer American blood donors, the numbers were quite similar (1 in 133, to be exact). In this latter study, conducted by Dr. Alessio Fassano of the University of Maryland, 1 out of 8 subjects identified as having celiac disease was African American. Given the small number of African Americans in the study sample, no definite conclusions could be made regarding the initial impression that the prevalence of celiac disease among this minority was similar to the prevalence described in Caucasians. And given the current state of awareness and testing, it is estimated that for each person diagnosed with celiac disease, there are seven who have not been identified yet!

Efforts to increase awareness about celiac disease are under way, and a significant number of support groups, research efforts, and specialty centers devoted to the diagnosis and management of this condition have been established. We hope this wave of information will sweep the country, leaving in its wake more informed families, doctors, nutritionists, and scientists. (See the appendix for the names of some of these organizations and support groups.)

Symptoms

As mentioned, symptoms of celiac disease can vary significantly. They may be prominent and debilitating and occur soon after exposure to gluten, or they may be subtle, so much so that they are only picked up because of a screening test or during the investigation of other conditions, such as slow growth or chronic headaches. Some people even carry genetic markers for the condition but never show symptoms. Most of the time, however, some symptoms are present. Any of the following in children and adolescents might indicate celiac disease:

- Chronic diarrhea
- Failure to thrive
- Weight loss
- Irritability
- Pallor and anemia
- Abdominal distension and excessive gassiness or bloating
- Bulky, foul-smelling stools
- Constipation
- Tooth discoloration and enamel breaks
- Joint and muscle pains
- Delayed onset of puberty
- Irregular menstrual periods

PERSONALITY CHANGES

Personality changes in children with celiac disease can be striking: these children can be clingy, easily upset, whiny, apathetic, or unusually sensitive and prone to tantrums. No one knows why exposure to the gluten proteins causes these behavioral changes. It has been suggested that part of their abnormal immune response affects the brain directly, or that by causing the intestine to be inflamed and damaged, certain toxins (perhaps from the bacteria that live in the gut) can get absorbed and cause changes in the chemistry of the brain. Amazingly, though, once the gluten-free diet starts, parents will report the most dramatic changes—"he's a different child," "can't recognize her"—as if, indeed, a poison had been taken away—which, technically, is what's happened!

Celiac disease seems to be a factor in other conditions as well. For example, calcium deposits have been found in brain scans of some celiac patients. Other celiac patients might experience recurrent seizures or sometimes show features of schizophrenia and bipolar disorders. How these conditions are related to gluten exposure, if indeed they are, or to the disturbed immunity caused by it remains a mystery and an area of active investigation.

Diagnosis

The gold standard for diagnosing celiac disease is still the examination of a sample of the small intestine. As described in chapter 5, small biopsies of the intestinal lining can easily be obtained at the time of an endoscopy, a test carried out under sedation or anesthesia. Parents always ask why they can't just try the gluten-free diet and see if their child gets better. This is a good question. Why put the child through the inconvenience and discomfort of an endoscopy if the response to being off all wheat products can show whether symptoms are connected to the diet? These are important reasons for recommending a biopsy. First, celiac disease is a diagnosis that affects the child's whole life and should not be made unless one is certain that the villi show the damage and the expected inflammation. In addition, improvement of symptoms when eliminating wheat and other cereals from the diet has been found in conditions where the intestine is not damaged at all. The gassiness and cramps these patients experienced might have been related to the way the cereal was broken down in the intestine. Similarly, some children might actually have a temporary allergy to wheat, like the temporary allergy other children may develop to dairy products or chicken, and in such cases, a lifelong avoidance of wheat would be unnecessary. And finally, simply adopting the gluten-free diet without a biopsy is not wise because if the diagnosis of celiac disease is made on the basis of improvement of symptoms, one might be tempted to reintroduce wheat at a later date or be less than strict about sticking to the diet. Either of these actions could cause serious health problems down the road. Hence, until someone develops a foolproof noninvasive test that is as reliable as the intestinal biopsy, we will need to continue trusting in the biopsy as the best diagnostic test for celiac disease.

Before a biopsy is considered, however, there are valuable blood tests that can be used to identify those with atypical symptoms or no symptoms at all. None of them are 100 percent reliable, but if they are positive and the biopsy confirms the diagnosis, the blood test can subsequently be used to monitor response to the diet and inadvertent exposure to gluten-containing food.

Treatment

Celiac disease is the only autoimmune disease for which we not only know the reason—gluten sensitivity—but also have a cure: the gluten-free diet. Celiac disease does not go away on its own, no matter how many times parents might hear about a relative or friend who "outgrew" the problem. It must be treated, and doing so effectively means following a strict gluten-free diet *for life*. Any amount of cheating is to be discouraged: the immune system does not need large amounts of gluten to be activated, even imperceptibly, and small, subtle exposures can do damage.

The Gluten-Free Diet

The initial response of a parent hearing a diagnosis of celiac disease and the need to start a gluten-free diet is one of horror: How can we possibly stick to this?! There is gluten everywhere! How is she going to manage in school? How is he going to handle cafeteria food or going to restaurants?

The gluten-free diet causes a major upheaval in the life of any child and his family. Fortunately, adaptation to the diet is, for the most part, painless. It is also very gratifying, for not only do parents see the changes occur in front of their eyes, but their "new child" reinforces the diet in a positive way. And with the help of knowledgeable nutritionists, dietitians, support groups, and the Internet, parents soon acquire a proficiency to match any of their physicians. (See appendix for details on these groups: many of the organizations provide gluten-free guides and cookbooks.)

In addition, many food companies make gluten-free products, and there is a wide variety of offerings: who would have thought of gluten-free pancakes, dinner rolls, pound cake, or pizza crust? Delicious snacks and exotic ethnic meals have relieved gluten-avoiders of the monotony of shopping and eliminated the feeling of being deprived or punished.

Once parents teach their children the ins and outs of the diet, the children often become their own best advocates, looking out for themselves in school or with friends. They know how to keep healthy and develop strategies so as to not feel bad about living with their diet restrictions. Of course, this does not happen overnight, and parents have to be prepared to expect complaints, expressions of frustration, and rebellion, but ultimately results seem to speak for themselves.

Reading labels becomes second nature to children and families with celiac disease, and they learn to recognize the places gluten can hide—it's in many food ingredients never identified as such! The following list gives just a few of the diet items to avoid:

Barley	Bran
Bulgur	Malt
Matzo meal	Rye
Soy (unless specifically gluten free)	Teriyaki sauce
Triticale (a hybrid of wheat and rye)	Wheat

The case against oats is not yet closed, and some studies suggest that the gluten in oats can be eaten without damaging the intestine. However, most dietitians in the United States still recommend avoiding oats altogether.

The gluten-free diet also applies to items such as toothpaste, vitamins, mineral supplements, and mouthwash. The watchword is, if you can ingest it, check to make sure it is safe to do so.

The celiac disease community has fought hard to shine more light on the possible hidden sources of gluten. Hopefully, this will continue to improve until the process is error proof. In the meantime, informed and vigilant reading of all labels will help identify some unexpected sources, among them foods we thought we could trust. To complicate matters, manufacturers sometimes change their ingredients without notice, thus introducing a possible wrench in a well-planned shopping routine. Toll-free numbers are always a good resource to call for updates or to clarify the possibility of gluten in any food item.

If you are going on a short trip, you are much less likely to have problems if you prepare your own food and bring it with you. When you eat out, many restaurants will be able to steer you toward safe dishes and many will accommodate reasonable requests. It always makes sense to call ahead to a restaurant to see if they are familiar with the gluten-free diet. Likewise with airlines: a gluten-free diet can be ordered ahead of time for most flights.

CHAPTER 16

Inflammatory Bowel Disease:
Ulcerative Colitis and Crohn's Disease

CHRONIC DIARRHEA . . . RECURRENT FEVERS . . .
FATIGUE . . . DELAYED GROWTH . . . NIGHT SWEATS

Inflammatory bowel disease (IBD) is the general term given to chronic inflammation of the intestines not caused by a known infection or other identifiable causes. IBD is the most noteworthy cause of chronic gastrointestinal (GI) disease, both in adults and children. It takes two forms, Crohn's disease (CD) and ulcerative colitis (UC). In this chapter, we will outline their similarities and differences and update your knowledge of these important conditions. We will also discuss the role of diet in treating IBD and how best to approach alternative and complementary therapies for children with IBD.

When I first saw Jeremy, he was fifteen and had been suffering from recurrent stomachaches as well as poor weight and height gain for two years. He had become very height conscious, as all his friends seemed to have grown taller than him, and he became even more frustrated when he compared his body to others in gym. Some of his friends were even starting to shave. Jeremy's parents suspected that he was not growing well because he did not eat nearly enough. But no matter how much Jeremy tried to eat, he felt full after a few bites. He preferred to eat small meals throughout the day, and he tried to eat healthy. Even so, he had terrible gas and frequent stomachaches. He was also unusually tired and had taken to napping in the afternoon before tackling homework. After examining Jeremy and completing his evaluation with blood tests, X-ray studies, and a colonoscopy, a diagnosis of Crohn's disease was confirmed.

The reason for focusing on IBD in some detail in this book is that it's often accompanied by stomachaches, but, unaware of this relationship, too many people endure a lot of unnecessary suffering as proper diagnosis is delayed. As we will show, many of IBD's manifestations mimic symptoms of other conditions, and they are thus often confused with or blamed on more innocent issues such as indigestion, food intolerance, or an intestinal virus. As much as possible, we want to avoid delays in treatment so that proper care can be provided before the disease has had a chance to progress.

It is estimated that between 700,000 and 1 million Americans suffer from either Crohn's disease or ulcerative colitis, and many of them are young: more then half of the cases appear during the teenage years or early twenties. A genetically transmitted condition, IBD appears to run in families—having a relative with IBD makes one ten times more at risk for the condition than the general population—and affects some ethnic groups more frequently than others. It is five times more common, for instance, among Ashkenazi Jews than in the population at large, and relatively prevalent among Eastern European

Caucasians. And while IBD is also encountered in African-American and Hispanic populations, it is quite rare among Asians.

Ulcerative Colitis and Crohn's Disease

To help you understand the differences between these two conditions, we will compare and contrast some of their clinical features.

The main differences between ulcerative colitis and Crohn's disease are that with ulcerative colitis, inflammation is limited to the lining of the large intestine, or colon, while in Crohn's disease, inflammation runs the length of the digestive tract and affects all layers of its lining.

Inflammation resulting from ulcerative colitis always starts at the rectum and extends further to various degrees. In the worst cases it involves the whole colon. The most common symptoms of ulcerative colitis include the following:

- Abdominal pain
- Diarrhea and bloody diarrhea
- Urgency and *tenesmus**
- Rectal bleeding
- Loss of appetite

---

*Tenesmus is a painful sensation of not being finished after a bowel movement is passed: the need to continue passing stool is perceived, even if no more stool needs to be evacuated. When tenesmus is present, we can assume there is inflammation of the rectum because this is the area where there are nerve endings that convey such a sensation.

- Weight loss
- Fatigue

As it affects the entire GI tract, Crohn's disease can involve the mouth, esophagus, stomach, and any part of the small or large bowel. Symptoms depend on which part of the intestines is inflamed. Most commonly, it is the juncture of the terminal ileum and cecum, or the area where the last segment of the small intestine meets the beginning of the colon. (Remembering the look of panic and desperation when mentioning the word "terminal" to one of my patients, I quickly add that here it just means "at the end of!") The most common symptoms of Crohn's disease are:

- Abdominal pain
- Intermittent diarrhea
- Fatigue
- Fevers and night sweats
- Poor weight gain and growth
- Delayed onset of puberty
- Poor appetite

The inflammation associated with Crohn's is responsible for the fevers and night sweats: it is a similar reaction to that found with other inflammatory conditions such as arthritis. Hence, night sweats and unexplained fevers should raise a red flag that should be addressed immediately. Diarrhea with Crohn's disease is intermittent; it might disappear for weeks, only to return unexpectedly, last for a few days or weeks, and clear up again. Such diarrhea is not necessarily bloody, as is the case in ulcerative colitis, unless the Crohn's involves the colon, in which case the symptoms might be very similar to those of ulcerative colitis. However, even Crohn's patients who do not have visible blood in their stool or diarrhea might develop iron deficiency from losing blood in minute amounts.

The poor weight gain and delayed growth in children and adolescents with Crohn's disease are directly related to poor appetite and insufficient caloric intake. When teenagers with Crohn's disease count their calories and keep a food diary, it's not unusual to find that they are eating a lot less than they should, so it's no wonder they don't grow: they are barely maintaining their weight and consuming only 60 to 70 percent of the calories they need. What causes this marked decrease in food intake? Simply put, kids avoid eating because it causes stomachaches and, at times, nausea. And inflammation suppresses the appetite as well.

The importance of measuring your child's weight and height regularly cannot be overemphasized, for this simple habit can help identify the first signs of a slowdown in growth. Sadly, we often encounter teenagers who look much younger than their age, for whom a red flag should have been raised years before. Because nearly 25 percent of patients with Crohn's develop the disease before adolescence, this is a valuable message: plot your child's height and weight growth on a chart. Either do it yourself or ask your health care provider to do it regularly.

It's Not Only in the Gut

Inflammatory bowel disease is a generalized immune disorder, meaning that despite its name, it is not confined to the digestive system. The immune system targets the intestine primarily, but other organs can come under attack. In fact, symptoms occur in other organs—most commonly the eyes, thyroid gland, skin, liver, joints, and kidneys—in one of four patients at some point in their illness. Interestingly, some of these symptoms can appear even before the intestine is affected and can remain active even after the inflammation of the intestine is under control.

Causes of IBD

Common medical wisdom now views IBD as a group of diseases caused by an abnormal immune response to internal as well as external triggers. We believe that the immune system of someone with IBD is genetically predisposed to overreact, injuring the intestinal tract and other organs. We still do not know for certain, however, what the exact reasons for this genetic predisposition are, nor have we determined the actual triggers sending the immune response careening out of control.

Complicating the riddle of IBD is that it is quite different from many other genetically determined disorders in which a defect or single gene at the root of the condition can be pinpointed. In IBD, several genes seem to be involved. Genetic research has moved forward noticeably with the completion of the Human Genome Project, however, and we can now offer hope to our patients and their families that a cure for IBD is in sight. The search continues at a feverish pace, and we expect to find answers in the next few years.

ENVIRONMENTAL FACTORS

For unknown reasons, inflammatory bowel disease is more common in areas of the world with better hygienic conditions and where parasitic and bacterial infections are relatively rare. In developing countries, populations routinely contract and over-come many intestinal infections. Does that somehow protect them against a misdirected immune response? If this turns out to be the case, then, ironically, IBD will have to be seen as an unintended consequence of the progress made in the control and eradication of infectious diseases!

Other environmental factors implicated in the development of IBD have included mycobacteria and the measles virus, each of which has been the subject of research. (Mycobacteria are the infectious agents responsible for various forms of tuberculosis.) Interestingly, the first descriptions of Crohn's disease—including those by its discoverers, Dr. Burrill Crohn and his colleagues—pointed out the similarities between the lesions it produced in the intestine and those caused by tuberculosis. Even under the micro-scope, the type of inflammation—with the presence of giant cells (granulomas)—and the changes in the wall of the intestine caused by Crohn's disease all resembled the effects of tuberculosis on the intestine. (Before the age of pasteurization, tuberculosis was a common infection of the bowel.) Since then, however, many med-ication trials using anti-TB drugs have failed to control IBD's effects, suggesting that an infection with mycobacteria is unlikely to be the cause of IBD.

Meanwhile, there has been an increased incidence of Crohn's disease in industrialized countries over the last sixty years. In 1995, British researchers reported epidemiological evi-dence connecting this spike with the eradication of the original measles virus after the institution of universal immunization programs using the modified (but still live) virus. Data revealed that Crohn's disease was five times more common in young adults at the end of 1990s than it had been in the 1970s: perhaps Crohn's disease was an inappropriate immune response to the measles vaccine by a predisposed individual.

This finding was very controversial, in no small part because it led many parents to stop immunizing their children against measles, and in turn there has since been a rise in the number of cases in Britain and elsewhere. However, the conclusions of the British study have not been borne out by other studies carried out in Europe and the United States.

STRESS AND OTHER PSYCHOLOGICAL FACTORS

Not surprisingly, the notion that IBD is caused by stress and strained family relations has thrived ever since Freud's psycho-analytical revolution. Certainly, any child (or adult) with a chronic disease that disrupts daily life routines and damages their self-esteem is going to be stressed, and now that we have begun to decipher some of the complex interaction between the mind and body, it is also becoming clear that stress does indeed play a role in immune-system function. However, we don't think that stress is what causes IBD, although once IBD develops, reduction of stress will help at many levels and should become an integral part of treatment.

Treatment of IBD: Today and Tomorrow

Fortunately, we have a whole array of medications to help bring inflammation under control and bring health back to those suffering from IBD. The goals in managing a child with IBD are not only to control inflammation but also to normalize nutritional status and replenish any nutritional deficiencies, ensure adequate growth and development, and provide guidance and support to maintain self-esteem.

The most commonly used drugs for the management of IBD include sulfasalazine and other similar aminosalicylic acid–containing products such as Asacol, Dipentum, Colazal, or Pentasa; steroid anti-inflammatory medicines such as prednisone or prednisolone may also be an option. In addition, immunosuppressants such as 6-mercaptopurine, azathioprine, and methotrexate and biological agents such as infliximab (Remicade) are extremely helpful for certain patients. Nutritional therapy, either as a primary treatment or as a complement to standard medications, continues to gain acceptance as well. Finally, the use of "good bacteria" (probiotics) is expanding and their proper role is still being defined through carefully conducted studies.

SULFASALAZINE

Sulfasalazine, the original and most widely prescribed medication for ulcerative colitis, was serendipitously developed in the 1940s by Nana Svartz, a Swedish rheumatologist. Dr. Svartz started treating her rheumatoid arthritis patients—the king of Sweden among them—with an aspirin-like anti-inflammatory attached to sulfapyridine, an antibiotic, thinking that the arthritis resulted from an infection and hoping that the aminosalicylic acid (ASA) of the aspirin would help to slow the antibiotic absorption and thus make it more effective. The combination, originally intended to treat arthritis, was found to be effective against colitis as well. However, its use was associated with such unpleasant side effects as nausea, rashes that

> broke out after exposure to the sun, and other allergic reactions. Twenty years after the drug was first used, it was discovered that the aminosalicylic acid component, the aspirin-like ingredient, was responsible for its beneficial effects; while the side effects were mostly caused by the sulfa-type antibiotic.

ASPIRIN-LIKE ANTI-INFLAMMATORY PREPARATIONS

After the experience with sulfasalazine (see sidebar on page 197), other methods of delivering the aminosalicylic acid (ASA) compound have been developed, including enteric coating the pills or microencapsulating the drug. A slow-release formulation, for example, makes it possible to maintain the action and diminish the side effects. Effective only in cases of mild to moderately severe inflammation, ASA preparations are particularly useful for maintenance of remission (the state of normalcy when symptoms are controlled and inflammation is low). For more severe attacks of IBD, steroids are a more powerful and faster-acting alternative.

STEROIDS

The steroids used in IBD are not the kind of anabolic steroids the public associates with building muscles and illegally enhancing sports performance. Nonetheless, a generalized fear of steroids is very real among certain caregivers, and there is reluctance to use them, even in circumstances when they might be the best choice for the patient.

In defense of caution, however, the list of possible side effects from steroids is long and frightening: diabetes, bone damage and osteoporosis, high blood pressure, acne, stretch marks, disfiguring weight gain, emotional changes, and a "moon" face, among others. No surprise, then, that anyone reading this list in a drug-information reference book would run away from steroids in a panic.

But don't panic! When used carefully, steroids are life-savers that provide us with a powerful weapon with which to contain the rampant inflammation that causes serious complications such as profuse bloody diarrhea and severe abdominal pain. They can also help prevent damage to eyesight when the immune response causes the eyes to be inflamed.

Steroids do, however, suppress growth, so we avoid using them for long periods. Yet we also know that poorly controlled IBD has serious side effects of its own, including malnutrition, anemia, intractable pain, and delayed growth. Therefore, the doctor's role is to use all available medications, including steroids if appropriate, to promote health, shorten the duration of the inflammation, and sustain remission. This is as much an art as it is a science. Individual patients respond differently to the same medications, and their IBD runs very different courses, some being very aggressive with repeated flare-ups while others are more subtle, with long periods of well-being. When we do prescribe steroids, it is for a short period, tapering off and phasing out the doses as quickly as possible and introducing in their place a second or third medication for long-term maintenance.

IMMUNOSUPPRESSANT DRUGS

Some of our best drugs for maintaining long-term remission of IBD are the immunosuppressant drugs such as 6-mercapto-

purine (6-MP), azathioprine, and methotrexate. These medications suppress the immune system's inflammatory response.
Now that we can measure the concentration of the active drug
in the blood they have proven to be very effective and much safer
to use than they were in the past. By keeping those levels within safe limits, potential side effects can be minimized or avoided
altogether.

REMICADE

Remicade (infliximab) is probably *the* major advance in the
management of IBD so far. Primarily used to treat Crohn's disease, it is the only medication that seems to change the natural
progression of the disease.

Remicade is an antibody against TNF-alpha (tumor necrosis factor alpha), one of the most important chemicals involved
in the intestinal inflammation of IBD, binding to it and neu-
tralizing its damaging effects. Remicade has also been successfully used in patients with rheumatoid arthritis and other
autoimmune disorders.

The clinical results of Remicade have been most dramatic in
patients suffering from extensive and intractable fistulas, which
are abnormal passages between adjacent organs. In cases of
Crohn's disease, a fistula might occur between an inflamed loop
of intestine and the bladder, or another loop of bowel, the
vagina, or even to the skin. In the past, fistulas were most difficult to treat and tended to recur, often causing a great deal of
misery. Remicade has been shown to help fistulas close effectively and definitively. For some patients, including teenagers,
regular use of Remicade (given intravenously for three hours,
every six to eight weeks) has been the only effective therapy for
their IBD. With such treatment, their quality of life has im-

proved immensely: they can lead normal lives again, free of recurrent surgeries and hospitalizations.

THE SURGICAL OPTION

In extreme circumstances, IBD patients may have to consider surgery to mitigate their condition.

The major indications for surgery in cases of *ulcerative colitis* are unremitting inflammation that is not responding to any treatment whatsoever and as prophylaxis against colon cancer. After ten years of living with ulcerative colitis, a person's risk of colon cancer increases by about 5 percent a decade. Regular surveillance by colonoscopy is indicated to identify colon cancer at its earliest stage. To avoid the possibility of colon cancer and cure ulcerative colitis, complete removal of the colon with a colectomy can be performed. The operation preserves the nerves and muscles of the rectum and, later, after a *pullthrough operation* (during which the small bowel is connected to the anus), the patient can be continent again and avoid the permanent use of an external bag.

The most common indications for surgery in *Crohn's disease* are bleeding, intractable pain, and intestinal obstruction. The latter is particularly troublesome because recurrent bouts of partial obstruction might be accompanied by distension, nausea, vomiting, weight loss, and lack of appetite, leading eventually to the passage becoming so narrow as to preclude normal nutrition.

A major difference between surgery in ulcerative colitis and in Crohn's disease is that while surgery cures ulcerative colitis, it is only a temporary measure in Crohn's disease. With Crohn's cases, we try to avoid surgery as long as the situation can be effectively managed with medications, because Crohn's disease tends to recur, usually at the site of the surgery. There is hope that maintaining patients with Crohn's on immunomodulatory medications after surgery will slow down, or perhaps altogether remove, the risk of recurrence.

THE DIETARY CONNECTION

The interest in nutrition as a means of enhancing health is nowhere as intense and controversial as when it targets chronic conditions for which there are no effective therapies. The idea that the immune system can be tamed or enhanced by adherence to certain diets is linked to the suspicion that the damage seen in inflammatory bowel disease is caused by certain items in the patient's diet.

Nutritionists, holistic practitioners, naturopaths, and other alternative-care providers have promoted some of these views without providing solid evidence to substantiate their claims. As a result, a dual system of care has evolved: the conventional system on the one hand, and the alternative or complementary one on the other.

Often parents are shy or embarrassed to confide in their doctor that they have visited or are following the recommendations of such practitioners. It is a pity, because that way we lose the opportunity to have an open and informative dialogue. I have not observed IBD sufferers gaining any particular benefits from diets restricted in wheat, dairy products, or refined sugars, but if any of my patients want to follow such diets—without hastily removing the anti-inflammatory medications that keep the disease under control, of course—we work together on a plan and discuss the details openly.

Notwithstanding the claims swirling around the Internet, there is no evidence that IBD is caused by a specific component of the diet, or that eliminating an item or items from the diet can result in a cure. Unfortunately, it's not that simple or straightforward. If any evidence for these guidelines existed, recommendations would have been agreed upon a long time ago.

This is not to say that the medical establishment completely disregards the role nutrition plays in the health of the intestine and in control of the immune system. On the contrary, we frequently use nutritional therapy to decrease inflammation and optimize growth in adolescents with delayed growth.

NUTRITIONAL SUPPLEMENTS

The use of liquid nutritional supplements has been associated with good clinical responses—meaning reduced inflammation—in patients with Crohn's disease. The results are almost comparable with those observed with a short course of steroids. An exclusively liquid diet somehow quiets down the immune system and decreases inflammation of the intestine. That much we know. The problem is that as soon as solid food is reintroduced, inflammation flares up again. Can you imagine staying on a liquid diet indefinitely? Neither can most Crohn's patients, so we use liquid nutritional supplements only as indicated, when needed, and for as long as practical.

ALTERNATIVE MEDICINE AND IBD

Parents and doctors tend to look at alternative and complementary medicines from different perspectives. It is part of a doctor's training to trust facts based on evidence, to ask for objective results obtained in controlled studies and under rigorous research conditions. Parents on the other hand sometimes accept ideas that correspond with or reinforce their own point of view on health and disease, attracted by general notions of "naturalness" and the perceived benefits of organic products.

To some extent, the Internet has created a wider gap between "them" and "us." Every wild theory and peculiar diet imaginable is to be found somewhere among the IBD links (of which there were over 200,000 in 2003). It sometimes bears reminding that just because something is on the Internet doesn't mean it's true. That is not to say that there is not a substantial amount of good and valuable information that can be found online, but parents must use their common sense.

You can visit the Crohn's and Colitis Foundation of America, the National Center for Complementary and Alternative Medicine of the National Institutes of Health, and other Web sites listed in the appendix for updated and scientifically sound and practical discussion of all aspects of IBD.

IBD Prognosis

When a child is diagnosed with inflammatory bowel disease, we can now discuss the disease with parents in a more positive manner than we would have been able to do fifteen years ago. Not only do we understand the disease better today, but thanks to the advances in molecular biology and genetics, we are at the threshold of being able to change its natural progression. Until that happens, we have excellent medications to manage the more severe attacks and effective maintenance drugs that can keep inflammation and the immune response at bay. A child with IBD probably will have to see a doctor more often than other kids, but good remissions can be maintained routinely.

Looking into the future, new and novel immune treatments will become available that will suppress the abnormal cells causing IBD and, for all intents and purposes, offer a cure. I'm optimistic!

CHAPTER 17

Helicobacter pylori, Ulcers, and Gastritis: How and When to Treat Them

HEARTBURN . . . NAUSEA . . . POOR APPETITE . . .
VOMITING BLOOD . . . PASSING BLACK, STICKY
STOOLS

While it might be fairly common knowledge that peptic ulcers are not caused by a bad diet, many people are still surprised to know that most duodenal ulcers are, in fact, products of an infectious disease. One of the major medical breakthroughs of the last twenty years has been the discovery that the vast majority of ulcers in the duodenum are caused by infection, and not stress, spicy foods, or alcohol.

H. Pylori Infection

The bacterium causing the infection is called *H. pylori,* or, more formally, *Helicobacter pylori.* The "helico" refers to the fact that the bacterium is shaped like a helix or a corkscrew, and this shape might help it to burrow through the protective mucus lining the stomach and settle deep in the tissues. Whether or not that is the case, *H. pylori* has nevertheless adapted to live in the stomach and duodenum. As *H. pylori* is mostly a disease of humans, the human intestine is where the organism resides. Accordingly, most infections are contracted through the oral-fecal or oral-oral route.

The stomach is what we would generally consider a hostile environment; the acid in it is capable of killing most of the yeast and bacteria we swallow. The fact that *H. pylori* has evolved to live and thrive in a place as acidic as the stomach is nothing short of amazing. *H. pylori* is found in all parts of the world, and it is estimated that in developing countries, anywhere from 3 to 10 percent of the population acquires the infection each year. In industrialized countries, the incidence is about 0.5 percent per year.

In this chapter, we will look at *H. pylori* infection in children and the role it plays in causing an inflammation of the stomach (gastritis) and duodenal ulcers. As *H. pylori* is not the only reason for gastritis, we will discuss its other causes and the treatments that are available to heal the inflammation.

What Is the Best Test?

There are three methods to test for *H. pylori:* endoscopy, blood tests, and the urea breath test. At present, the only reliable way to identify the presence of gastritis or an ulcer due to *H. pylori* is to perform an endoscopy (see chapter 5) and locate the bacterium with special stains (a culture is not routinely done).

The blood tests currently available to test for *H. pylori* are not reliable enough in determining whether the infection is present. The results are difficult to interpret, and we'd have to decide whether to treat a child with presumed, not conclusively diagnosed, infection.

Likewise, more research is needed before we can depend fully on the urea breath test as a means of pinpointing *H. pylori* infection in children. Should it eventually prove effective, the urea test will be a very good noninvasive diagnostic tool. A proven application of the urea breath test is in confirming that the infection has cleared after treatment. This avoids having to perform another endoscopy if the child relapses or if symptoms persist after treatment.

MEDICAL PIONEERS

The story behind the identification of *H. pylori* as the cause for many ulcers is extraordinary. Working in Perth, Australia, in the early 1980s, doctors J. Robin Warren and Barry Marshall thought that they found a link between the bacterium and ulcers. Their thesis was met with a great deal of skepticism and opposition.

Dr. Marshall followed an unconventional route to prove that he was right. In 1984, he infected himself by swallowing enough *H. pylori* bacteria to make himself ill. Indeed, he developed gastritis, an inflamed stomach lining, and had it confirmed through an endoscopy.

The medical community eventually accepted the implications of Barry Marshall's experiment. But, it was not until 1994 that a National Institutes of

**Health conference fully vindicated Marshall,
releasing a statement confirming that *H. pylori*
causes ulcers.**

To Treat or Not to Treat

When both inflammation and *H. pylori* organisms are found in
the same endoscopic biopsy, the condition is deemed an active
H. pylori infection. Only active infections identified by
endoscopy should be treated, so as not to expose the child
unnecessarily to a great deal of medication for several weeks.
The treatments for *H. pylori* are not effective for other ailments,
so care focuses on children with proven active *H. pylori* conditions, those with flattening of the stomach lining and *H. pylori*
infection, as well as children with a past history of stomach or
duodenal ulcers in whom active *H. pylori* is proven. Cases in
which the presence of an ulcer is diagnosed with certainty by X-
ray film as part of an upper GI series (see chapter 5) also deserve
treatment.

Decisions about treatment in cases of gastritis without duodenal ulcers are more difficult, even when *H. pylori* has been
identified in the tissues by biopsy because the results do not
always turn out to be curative. There are several good reasons to
treat, however. Among them is the hope that getting rid of the
infection will help prevent the development of ulcers, that stomachaches will improve, and that flattening of the stomach lining
may be avoided.

Successful treatment of *H. pylori* depends on ensuring that
all medication is taken regularly and consistently. This may go
without saying, but when the treatment involves taking three or

four different medications two or three times a day for two or three weeks, compliance becomes a real issue with children (and with many adults also!).

Treatment is effective in eradicating the infection in 80 to 85 percent of cases, but some strains of *H. pylori* have become resistant to particular antibiotics. Treatment is also compromised when the patient has received medication to decrease acidity before starting therapy.

All these issues point to the need for caution when treating patients with abdominal pain from suspected gastritis. The idea is to avoid overtreatment that might expose children to repeated courses of unnecessary antibiotics.

Symptoms of Gastritis and Ulcers

Children with an inflammation of their stomach or duodenum will often experience abdominal pain. Typically, this pain improves after eating, but not as consistently among children as adults. Unlike adults, children with gastritis or ulcers do not tend to wake up in the middle of the night experiencing heartburn or a piercing stomachache. More commonly, their pain from gastritis is centered over the pit of the stomach, comes and goes, and might be accompanied by additional symptoms, including nausea and vomiting, loss of appetite, weight loss, bloating and feeling full all the time, and excessive gas

RED FLAGS

Some symptoms require immediate medical attention because they indicate that an ulcer has gone so deep as to perforate, or break through the wall of the stomach or intestine. Medical attention should be sought immediately in cases of sudden, persistent, and worsening stomach pain, repeated vomiting, bloody or black, sticky stools (melena), and blood in the vomit.

Vomiting may occur when an ulcer affects the duodenum, causing it to spasm, swell, and become blocked. If the vomit contains bright-red blood, the ulcer has eroded into a blood vessel. If the vomit appears to have coffee grounds in it, that is digested blood—signifying bleeding. In either situation, do not wait. *Call your doctor immediately!* Although, in many cases the bleeding stops on its own, blood in the vomit can be a major emergency.

If blood from a duodenal ulcer moves through the intestine, it turns black and sticky by the time it comes out in the stool. The smell of digested blood is quite disgusting. This particular type of stool is called melena, and it is an important red flag, as it implies bleeding from the upper gastrointestinal tract.

Stress Ulcers

Stress-related ulcers are *not* caused by day-to-day tension or worry, but by conditions of medical distress. When there is diminished blood flow to the intestinal organs, it disrupts the protective mucus barrier, rendering the intestinal wall vulnerable. This typically happens when a patient is in shock because of bleeding or during severe infections when there are toxins in the blood. Stress ulcers also occur in patients who have undergone brain surgery, those with serious burns, and those who have suffered strokes.

Treatment is preventive. Effective acid suppression with intravenous or oral medications can help prevent stress ulcers in susceptible patients.

Gastritis Symptoms

Symptoms and manifestations of gastritis are similar whether *H. pylori* is involved or not. Children will complain of abdominal pains and nausea; they might lose their appetite and vomit. They might also lose weight or belch frequently.

In addition to *H. pylori*, other causes of gastritis include the use of nonsteroidal anti-inflammatory drugs (NSAIDs) like ibuprofen and aspirin, other medications, and alcohol.

DIAGNOSIS

Only through endoscopy can a diagnosis of gastritis be made with certainty. The findings from X-ray films are not specific, unless there is a clear ulcer crater. The radiologist might report irregularity of the lining, excess fluid in the stomach, or irregular contractions (spasm), but that is not enough to confirm the diagnosis.

TREATMENT

To treat gastritis, we recommend avoiding exposure to the irritants that caused it, whether aspirin or any other particular medication. Effective acid suppression is possible with the excellent medications at our disposal, which work to allow the lining of the stomach to regenerate and heal itself.

Allergic Gastritis

In children, the protective property of the stomach lining can be damaged by acid in combination with various irritants. This kind of gastritis can be caused by food allergies, and its hallmark is the presence of *eosinophils* in the biopsies. An eosinophil is a type of white cell that participates in many of the body's immune-related allergic reactions. For example, the mucus in the nose of someone suffering from pollen allergy is packed with eosinophils. Eosinophils contain small granules rich in histamine and other chemicals capable of expanding blood vessels and generating excess acidity. By disrupting the mucus barrier in the intestine they can open the door to inflammation. When this happens, the condition is named *eosinophilic gastritis.*

SYMPTOMS

Symptoms of eosinophilic gastritis include abdominal pains in infants, vomiting, and poor weight gain. The symptoms of food intolerance are hard to separate from those seen in gastro-esophageal reflux: many babies will be treated for acid reflux for weeks or months without full control of their symptoms. Not until an endoscopy is performed and biopsies reveal abnormal concentrations of eosinophils in the lining of the stomach (and sometimes in the esophagus and the duodenum) will the diagnosis be made correctly.

TREATMENT

Treatment of eosinophilic gastritis consists of avoiding the offending protein. Special hypoallergenic formulas are available for infants and are very effective in managing this type of gastritis. Normally, the immune system matures and, by the time a child is two or three years old, most allergic intestinal inflammations resolve.

However, eosinophilic gastritis can develop at any point beyond the early years, in which case it is usually a manifestation of a food allergy and hyperactive immune system. In more severe cases, steroids need to be used to control the inflammation.

CHAPTER 18

Cyclic Vomiting Syndrome

RECURRENT SEVERE VOMITING . . . NAUSEA . . .

LETHARGY . . . DEHYDRATION . . . MIGRAINES

Cyclic vomiting syndrome (CVS) is a relatively new diagnosis that is not yet widely recognized. Efforts are under way to increase the awareness of this particular type of vomiting, as it is easily confused with vomiting associated with viruses or food poisoning until one realizes that its pattern is both different and characteristic.

In fourteen-year-old Randy's case, it was the third visit to the emergency room, and the story had become all too familiar. He was retching, heaving, and vomiting every time he opened his eyes. He seemed to be in major distress. When he wasn't being sick, he preferred to sleep, lying in the fetal position. Noise seemed to particularly bother him, and the ride to the hospital had been a nightmare. The doctor asked the familiar questions: How long has this been going on? Has anyone else been sick at home? Did he have a fever? Did he have diarrhea with the vomiting? When was the last time he was able to urinate?

The answers to those questions about Randy's case history revealed his parents to be just as puzzled as his treating physicians in previous trips to the emergency room. Short hospitalizations had produced only an inconclusive diagnosis. The discharge papers always read "gastroenteritis" or "intestinal flu." The situation was even more frustrating because Randy had undergone extensive tests over the last year, including a head MRI, endoscopy of the stomach, an upper GI series, and a multitude of blood and urine tests. He had been seen by pediatric surgeons, neurologists, gastroenterologists, and even a child psychiatrist, who had been called in because there was no denying that several of Randy's episodes had occurred during what the consultant considered "stressful circumstances."

Through it all, Randy was an excellent student who never seemed to mind having to take exams and enjoyed a fun-filled social life in school. In fact, this last episode occurred during the ride to the airport on the way to a family vacation, and the previous one had taken place at a fabulous birthday celebration where there were clowns and magicians and Randy had been one of the "volunteers."

Randy's presentation, as it turned out, was typical of what is called cyclic vomiting syndrome (CVS).

Cyclic vomiting syndrome patients are distinguished by their perfect health between their periodic vomiting cycles and suffer no underlying conditions of any sort—intestinal obstructions or irritation, gallstones, and even brain tumors. Another feature of CVS is the unusually intense way in which the vomiting occurs. It is not unusual for the child to vomit every fifteen minutes and for these episodes to last for hours, sometimes days—one to four days is most common. Though the features of the vomiting episodes may vary from one child to the next, each child tends to develop his or her own repetitive pattern. CVS can start at any age, but it most often begins between the ages of three and seven. Adults can also develop this pattern of vomiting out of the blue, but for them, episodes tend to be less frequent, though they might last longer.

The picture of a child in a full blown CVS attack is quite frightening. The retching is long and drawn out and often produces green bile and sometimes even bloody mucus, due to the severity of the nausea. As a result, dehydration tends to occur. Even though some patients will feel incredibly thirsty and try to drink while retching and vomiting, they cannot keep the fluids down.

The child will also often complain of abdominal pains, which are usually severe enough to make everybody wonder whether the attack is due to acute appendicitis, a kidney stone, or an intestinal obstruction. He will often lie in the fetal position, trying to avoid interaction with the surrounding environment. In addition, teenagers, who are better able to talk about their experience than younger children, typically describe a sense of being out of their body; indeed mental changes during CVS episodes have been described as being in a "conscious coma." During the attack, too, adrenaline seems to be overflowing, inducing changes in blood pressure, pallor or a flushed appearance, chills or hot flashes, and goose bumps.

Four Common Phases

CVS is characterized by four phases that patients typically experience.

1. **PRODROME**   This phase, which can last from a few minutes to several hours, signals that a vomiting episode is about to start; a bellyache can be the very first sign. Taking medication at this point might stop an episode from developing. (Sometimes, however, an episode will start with no warning.)

2. **EPISODE**   This is the phase of intense vomiting and nausea. The child will be unable to eat or drink without vomiting, and he will be pale and drowsy, become exhausted, and go into a withdrawn state.

3. **RECOVERY**   The nausea and vomiting will finally stop, and the child's color, appetite, and energy will return.

4. **SYMPTOM-FREE INTERVAL**   This period can last from weeks to months.

Triggers

Episodes of CVS tend to happen when the child is excited (positively *or* negatively) or is overtired, or when the body is fighting an infection. The idea that CVS attacks are related to stress is supported by research by Dr. Yvette Tache of CURE: Digestive Disease Research Center at the West Los Angeles Veterans Administration Medical Center. Dr. Tache's work shows that an overproduction of, or abnormally acute sensitivity to, stress hormones produced by the brain plays an important role in triggering the CVS chain reaction. For example, new information has shown that the early-morning attacks typical of CVS coincide with a surge in corticotrophin releasing factor (CRF), a brain hormone that influences our circadian rhythm, or night-and-day cycles. This knowledge raises hope that CVS might someday be managed with CRF-blocking medications.

CVS and Migraine

Of great interest has been the realization that as children outgrow CVS—and more than 60 percent do—they will develop typical migraines. Characteristics common to CVS attacks and migraines include their relation to stress, hypersensitivity to noise and light, nausea, and vomiting. Furthermore, many factors that trigger CVS episodes also cause migraines, including certain food products like chocolate or aged cheeses. Not surprisingly, patients with CVS will find relief from medications that prevent or treat migraines.

Diagnosis

Diagnosing CVS remains difficult because it is still a relatively unfamiliar condition: many people do not recognize the pattern because they are simply unaware. There is no specific test that points directly to the right diagnosis, and doctors still rely on recognition of the recurrent pattern to identify CVS. In the last several years, however, many publications and presentations to health care professionals have increased awareness and understanding of the underlying triggers and mechanisms. CVS exemplifies a true brain-gut disorder, in which the disturbance in the brain's hormonal balance results in an escalation of nausea and vomiting involving the enteric nervous system, the brain in the gut.

Management

The watchword when treating a child with CVS is support: prevent dehydration and avoid the irritation that occurs as stomach acids are repeatedly brought up through the esophagus and mouth. If dehydration and its attendant salt and acid imbalance can be addressed early in a CVS episode, the duration of the attack may be shortened. During the full onset of an episode, this is accomplished by placing the patient in a quiet room and providing him with an intravenous glucose drip, as well as sedation.

Many parents of CVS-afflicted children have found it useful to carry a "CVS letter." Such a letter contains a brief description of the condition as well as providing a recommended protocol to address the nausea, pain, and need for fluid replacement. The letter also furnishes helpful instructions for managing the episode correctly and safely, and lists telephone contacts for physicians to call for more information. However, we can't forget that a child with CVS can, at some point, develop appendicitis or have another explanation for their vomiting attack!

The future will witness a major growth in our understanding of this mysterious and debilitating condition. What used to be considered psychological is now a prime example of problems that affect the brain, gut, and all of the relay stations in between.

CHAPTER 19

Pancreatitis

NAUSEA . . . VOMITING . . . FEVER . . . YELLOW
DISCOLORATION OF SKIN AND EYES . . .
GALLSTONES

As bellyaches go, the ones caused by pancreatitis, an inflammation of the pancreas, rank high among the most severe a child can experience. Fortunately, not all instances of pancreatitis are very acute, so the pain can be milder, mimicking the stomach flu or food indigestion.

The pancreas is a gland that sits against the vertebral column behind the stomach, hugged by the sweep of the duodenum. Because of its position, the pancreas is protected, yet also prone to damage: if there is blunt trauma to the abdomen, the pancreas can get crushed against the pillar of vertebrae right behind it.

The pancreas plays a vital role in the digestion of food. One of its two main functions is to produce the enzymes that we need to break down protein, fat, and starches. It is one of the marvels of our body that these powerful digestive enzymes, capable of dissolving protein and other complex foodstuffs, do not cause the pancreas to digest itself, but under normal circumstances, the pancreas is protected because it produces the enzymes in a form that is not active until they come into contact with food in the intestine at the time of digestion. When there is inflammation in the pancreas, however, activation can take place in the pancreas itself. Once this happens, the pancreas literally *can* eat itself away! This is why pancreatitis can be such a serious medical problem.

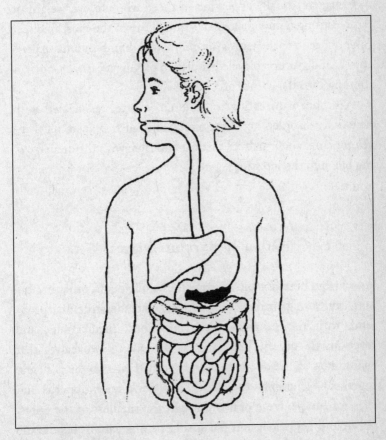

FIGURE #15   Location of the Pancreas

Causes: Acute and Chronic

Pancreatitis may be characterized as acute or chronic. Acute pancreatitis develops suddenly, lasts for a short period, and usually resolves completely. It can be caused by viruses or from a blockage of the pancreatic duct by a gallstone. Although gallstones are rare in young children, we do occasionally discover them through ultrasounds performed while evaluating problems completely unrelated to the gallbladder. They are more common in teenagers, usually appearing in those who are overweight or have a strong family history of stones. One of the most frequent cases of acute pancreatitis in children is blunt trauma experienced falling over a bicycle handlebar, playing a contact sport, or running into the corner of a table.

Chronic pancreatitis in children is often associated with hereditary disorders and certain problems, such as anatomical developmental abnormalities that can interfere with the drainage of the bile into the intestine.

Other Important Triggers

Aside from heredity and damage to the bile ducts, other important causes of pancreatitis in children include structural problems with the pancreas itself, infections, medications, and reactions to surgery. The pancreas is made of two halves that swing around the duodenum and meet, their two ducts fusing together. Sometimes the two halves don't fuse properly, and most of the pancreas drains through the smallest of the ducts. As a child gets older and the small opening cannot handle the larger volumes draining from the organ, a bottleneck will develop, and inflammation will result. In these cases, endoscopy (see chapter 5) will not only provide a proper diagnosis but also allow for widening of the duct. By enlarging the outlet, pancreatic juices will drain more normally and the pressure buildup is relieved.

Pancreatitis may also be brought on by viruses and other infections. The best-known infection that can cause pancreatitis in children is the mumps. The mumps virus causes inflammation of the parotid glands—the salivary glands in the face—and also of the pancreas and testicles. Mumps is now very rare in the United States because of the MMR vaccine, but unimmunized children in other parts of the world still regularly contract it. Other viruses, such as the hepatitis viruses, the Epstein-Barr virus (which causes mononucleosis), and various upper-respiratory or intestinal viruses can also cause mild pancreatitis.

In other cases, exposure to medications is the culprit for pancreatitis. The list of medications that can cause pancreatitis is long. The inflammation seems to be an allergic-type reaction in some cases, although in others damage occurs only after exceeding a certain dosage.

Pancreatitis after surgery is seen particularly after scoliosis repair. The reason is unclear; perhaps the inflammation is set off by manipulation of the spine or by the changes in the blood flow to the pancreas when the spine is straightened.

As mentioned, pancreatitis can be hereditary. An increased likelihood of pancreatitis is seen in certain inherited conditions, including mutations of the cystic fibrosis (CF) gene. Patients don't have full-blown cystic fibrosis, but they may suffer from recurrent pancreatitis. (For more information on other reasons for hereditary pancreatitis, see the appendix, pp. 243–46.)

Symptoms

The most common symptoms of pancreatitis include abdominal pain (typically at the pit of the stomach and back) as well as lack of appetite, nausea, and vomiting. The inflammation can also be accompanied by fever, and in the most severe cases, it can progress to shock. Dehydration is an issue as a result of the vomiting and fluid collection in the intestine. Management in an intensive-care unit is routine for the more severe cases of pancreatitis.

Diagnosis

When pancreatitis is suspected in a child with abdominal pains, blood tests are performed looking for abnormal levels of two important pancreatic enzymes: amylase and lipase. High levels of these enzymes in the blood indicate an ongoing inflammation in the pancreas. Confirmation that the pancreas is inflamed and swollen is made by a CT scan or a sonogram (see chapter 5). These tests are very sensitive and can also help identify stones, dilatation of the ducts, cysts, or abscesses.

Treatment

Managing the child with pancreatitis is supportive, focusing on pain control, rehydration, nutritional support, bowel rest, and, if necessary, drainage of cysts or abscesses.

Pancreatitis is not an oddity in the pediatric patient, so we will as a matter of course screen a child presenting with severe abdominal pain, nausea, and vomiting for this condition. Valuable diagnostic tests are available to pinpoint, and in many cases remove, the reason for the inflammation.

CHAPTER 20

Liver Diseases: What Are Jaundice, Hepatitis, and Cirrhosis in Children?

The American Liver Foundation estimates that as many as twenty-five million Americans have or have had some form of liver disease, including problems with the gallbladder and bile ducts. Although some causes of liver disease are rare among children and adolescents, there are many conditions that do affect them. Some of these are hereditary, and they appear at birth or shortly thereafter. Others are caused by viruses that can be contracted at any age. Liver problems range in severity from simple jaundice resulting from the immaturity of a baby's system to different types of hepatitis that pose serious short- and long-term consequences.

The liver is located on the right side of the chest, hidden under the ribs and protected by them. Only when the liver is enlarged can it be felt under the rib margin, but we can "listen" for it: by tapping on the ribs and listening for dullness, we can find out how large it has grown. (It's the same principle wine-makers use when they tap a barrel to find out how full it is.)

The liver is an extremely adaptable and resilient organ, capable of regenerating itself even after major injury. In some cases, however, the liver can malfunction completely—resulting in end-stage liver disease and failure. Major advances, including liver transplantation, however, have made this once-lethal condition one with a more hopeful and positive outlook.

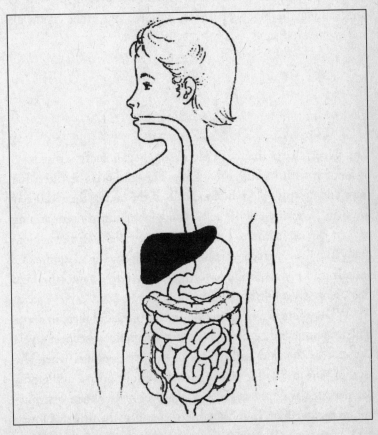

FIGURE #16   Location of the Liver

Liver Function

In chapter one, we described some of the important tasks carried out by the liver. It is a waste-treatment plant, a recycling center, and an amazing chemical factory; in a pinch, it can even act as a lunch counter. Among the liver's jobs are maintaining the body's metabolism and making bile, cholesterol, and clotting factors. It also manufactures glycogen, regulates the body's sugar balance, synthesizes fats, proteins, carbohydrates, and albumin, and stores vitamins, amino acids, and iron. Finally, the liver is responsible for cleaning the blood of toxins, poisons, and other chemicals and waste products.

Jaundice

The spleen shares the liver's blood supply and is often discussed in tandem with its larger neighbor. The spleen is the filter that traps and destroys old red blood cells at the end of their 120-day life span. It repackages the cells' hemoglobin, the iron-containing oxygen carrier in them, into a substance called *bilirubin*. Normally, the liver extracts this bilirubin from the circulation, converts it into a water-soluble form, and excretes it into the bile: that's what gives bile its green color.

When there is a malfunction in this process, bilirubin accumulates and jaundice develops. Visible jaundice—seen in a yellow cast to the skin and whites of the eyes—occurs when the level of bilirubin in the blood goes above four or five milligrams per deciliter, well above the normal level of less than one milligram per deciliter. In most cases of jaundice, the urine will turn dark, sometimes as dark as tea or cola.

Newborn jaundice, one of the most common and benign forms of jaundice, is caused by liver immaturity. Many newborn babies' livers cannot process bilirubin properly, allowing it to accumulate and lend the skin and eyes a yellowish tinge. The liver matures quickly, however, and the jaundice clears up by the time the child is one or two weeks old, though it might take a little longer in breast-fed infants. Often, the process is helped by exposure to light—either sunlight or special phototherapy lights in the hospital nursery or at home—which break down the bilirubin so that the body can excrete it. Doctors check the bilirubin levels in all newborns and decide whether it is safe to discharge them home or keep them in the hospital to wait for the levels to stabilize or decrease. When bilirubin is at a high level in the blood, it can reach the brain and cause damage.

Cirrhosis in Children

Even with approximately 20 percent of its cells working, the liver retains the capacity to sustain its important manufacturing and cleansing functions. Should more than 80 percent of the organ be damaged, however, the remaining liver might not be able to compensate any longer. At that point, the loss of liver function is very rapid and liver failure can develop unexpectedly.

When liver cells are inflamed, they die, and that sometimes causes scarring called *cirrhosis*. As scar tissue forms, it replaces the normal liver tissue, and when this happens, the scaffolding of connective tissue forming the frame that keeps all of the liver cells in place collapses. This results in poor blood filtration through the liver. Consequently, the spleen enlarges and internal bleeding can occur. This condition is called *portal hypertension*.

CAUSES OF CIRRHOSIS

Usually, people associate the term "cirrhosis" with alcohol. Certainly, excessive alcohol consumption is one of the leading causes of cirrhosis in adults, but children can have cirrhosis too and, in their case, it has nothing to do with drinking alcohol.

Children can develop cirrhosis as a result of congenital disorders. Sometimes, the lack of any one of a number of enzymes can allow the formation and buildup of damaging chemicals. In other situations, such as biliary atresia, bile cannot be pumped out of the liver because the bile ducts are not fully developed. This accumulation of bile in the liver is by itself damaging and promotes cirrhosis.

The most common childhood genetic diseases presenting with jaundice are alpha-1 antitrypsin deficiency, biliary atresia, galactosemia, hemochromatosis, hereditary fructose intolerance (HFI), and ornithine transcarbamilase (OTC) deficiency.

Only biliary atresia will be discussed in some detail because it is the most common chronic liver disease leading to transplantation.

Biliary Atresia

Biliary atresia, which literally means closure or absence of the bile channel or channels, is caused by the destruction of the bile ducts inside and outside the liver. This is a congenital disorder that affects one in twenty thousand live births and affects infants. The damage is progressive, but can be slowed down if diagnosis is made before the age of twelve weeks and surgery is successful.

Progression is variable, but without surgery all children die before age three. Even with surgery, however, many children with biliary atresia will eventually require liver transplantation. Fortunately, results have been excellent.

Infants with biliary atresia have no symptoms. They are usually healthy, full-term newborns who seem to be doing well, until a parent or health care provider notices a persistently yellow tint of the eyes and skin. Often, this is confused with normal newborn jaundice, delaying recognition of the real problem.

An important sign that helps distinguish between "normal" jaundice and something more serious—such as biliary atresia—is the color of the baby's stool. Bile makes the stool appear golden yellow to greenish, so stool that color is the best indicator that there is no obstruction and bile is getting through the ducts. Rather than being alarmed by green stools, parents should be very happy when they see their infant produce them: it is a reassuring sign. *Parents should call their physician immediately, however, if the stool is white or pale.*

Biliary atresia requires highly specialized surgery to correct. In the procedure, a loop of intestine is fashioned in such a way that it allows the bile to drain directly from the liver into the intestine. Babies who undergo this surgery require continued lifelong monitoring by the pediatrician and specialist: they will need fat-soluble vitamin supplements, any infection to be treated immediately, and the blood monitored regularly. Everyone must work to ensure that the baby is thriving.

If the disease progresses, children will develop portal hypertension, a sign that scar tissue is forming in the liver. Management of the complications of portal hypertension is left to the pediatric gastroenterologist.

Liver Transplant

Liver transplantation has come a long way in the forty years since it began; today's expected survival rate is 90 percent. The availability of living-donor programs allows the transplant to take place before the child's general health has deteriorated. Donor livers can also be split, allowing two children to get one portion each.

LIVER TRANSPLANT

Dr. Thomas Starzl performed the first liver transplant at the University of Colorado, in Denver, in 1963. The patient rejected the organ and died soon after. Four years later, however, in 1967, Dr. Starzl went on to successfully transplant a liver, using steroids and immunosuppression to combat rejection. That same year, in South Africa, Dr. Christiaan Barnard performed the world's first heart transplant.

Another groundbreaking milestone in transplant technique occurred in 1989 at the University of Chicago, with the first living-donor liver transplant: Alyssa Smith, an infant from Texas, received a portion of her mother's liver. The surgery was performed by Dr. Christoph Broelsch and Dr. Jean Emond.

Hepatitis

Hepatitis is a broad term that means inflammation of the liver. When most people hear the word "hepatitis," they think of a viral infection, most likely a contagious one. Yet while the cause can indeed be a viral infection, that is not the only possibility: hepatitis actually refers to any condition in which the liver cells are inflamed. We will discuss the viral forms first.

Viral Hepatitis

Viral hepatitis can be caused by any one of the many "alphabet" viruses: A, B, C, D, and so on, named in the order in which they were discovered. It can be acute or chronic, with some viral forms progressing from acute to chronic conditions and others never doing so. Hepatitis A, for example, is always acute and never becomes chronic, while hepatitis B will become chronic. Only the immune response of the patient determines whether or not the viral infection will be completely eliminated: there are no medications or diets that can prevent the conversion of an acute hepatitis infection into a chronic one. However, if the infection does become chronic, there are medications available to help the body abolish the virus.

Many hepatitis-causing viruses spread in unsanitary conditions. The virus is shed in the stool of infected people, and in areas of low sanitation, it can easily contaminate food or water. Anyone who eats or drinks contaminated food or water will contract the disease. Other forms of viral hepatitis can be passed through bodily secretions, including blood, and through sexual contact and intravenous drug use. Mothers can pass the virus to their babies during childbirth.

SYMPTOMS

Symptoms of viral hepatitis vary significantly from virus to virus and from patient to patient. Common symptoms, however, include abdominal pain and nausea, fatigue, loss of appetite and weight loss, jaundice, and dark urine or pale stools.

The pain children complain about when they have contracted hepatitis is usually vague, dull but steady, and located over the area of the liver in the right upper quadrant of the torso. It may also be felt in the center of the belly. Though many people associate the two, hepatitis and jaundice are not always related. We see cases of hepatitis where there is no jaundice and cases of jaundice where there is little hepatitis.

DIAGNOSIS

When symptoms indicate that hepatitis might be present, diagnosis of the type of infection and the extent of the inflammation will be confirmed and monitored by blood tests.

IMMUNIZATION

Impressive progress has been made in the last decade toward protecting our children against hepatitis A and hepatitis B. In 1996, hepatitis A vaccination was recommended for all children living in populations with the highest hepatitis A rates, which included American Indian, Native Alaskan, and selected Hispanic, migrant, and some religious communities. Later, the recommendation was extended to children living in states or counties with rates at least twice the national average for 1987 through 1997 (20 cases per 100,000 population). At present, the American Academy of Pediatrics recommends vaccinating all children in the United States against hepatitis A starting at age two. You should consult your child's health care provider for more information.

Since the guidelines for screening all expecting mothers for hepatitis B were implemented, there has been a sustained decrease in the occurrence of hepatitis B in children. Infants can develop chronic hepatitis B by contracting the infection from their mothers at birth, but now, when a mother is found to be a hepatitis B carrier, the infant will be given immunoglobulin shortly after birth and will be protected by a series of immunizations.

Hepatitis A

Hepatitis A tends to be a short-lived and self-limited infection, which means that even without treatment, the body will eliminate the infection, usually within one to two months. In children, the inflammation can be so mild that parents might not even detect its presence. If discovered, it is usually revealed when a blood test identifies antibodies against this virus in the blood. It should be noted that in very rare cases hepatitis A can run a very severe and sometimes even fatal course.

SYMPTOMS

A child will contract hepatitis A by putting contaminated objects in his or her mouth. It will not present right away, though, as it has an incubation period of three to four weeks. When symptomatic, it will present with vague complaints of tiredness, abdominal pain, lack of appetite, and nausea. Because these complaints are so common among children as to not raise an immediate red flag, some of the largest outbreaks tend to happen in nurseries and day care centers. (Teenagers—and adults—who smoke might describe a sudden aversion to cigarettes, which can be an early telltale sign of the infection.) By the time jaundice surfaces, the child is usually not infectious any longer. The virus is shed in the stool, another reason for its prevalence in large-group child-care situations.

The inflammation runs its course in three to six weeks and, unlike hepatitis B or C, never becomes chronic.

TREATMENT

Other than observing your child carefully and making sure she is eating and drinking well, there is no specific treatment for hepatitis A. In cases where there is significant weight loss, nutritional supplements may be called for. While the infection is active, we recommend that the child use her own plates, cutlery, toothbrushes, and other personal items, and do so until completely recovered.

HEPATITIS A VIRUS (HAV)	
TRANSMISSION	Infected body waste—to-oral contamination: not washing hands after changing the diaper of an infected child or going to the bathroom (if contaminated); through an infected food preparer; drinking contaminated water; or eating contaminated food, raw fish, and shellfish
AFFECTED POPULATIONS	People sharing food or facilities with infected individuals: day care, camp, school
PRESENTATION	Either mild symptoms or acute, flulike illness, with fever, nausea, vomiting, abdominal pain, diarrhea, jaundice, weight loss, and dehydration
CHRONIC?	No; does not usually last longer than six months
TREATMENT	Usually resolves itself in three to six weeks

HEPATITIS B

Hepatitis B is a more serious infection than hepatitis A because it can develop into a chronic form. When a child is infected with the hepatitis B virus at birth, the disease becomes chronic in 90 percent of cases.

The reason hepatitis B becomes chronic is that the virus insinuates itself into the DNA of the liver cells. When that happens, every time a liver cell divides, the virus divides with it. Sometimes the body cannot make antibodies against the virus so it cannot get rid of the infection.

Chronic hepatitis B is associated with a high rate of cirrhosis and liver cancer. In some parts of the world, the incidence of liver cancer is thirty to fifty times higher than in the general global population because of long-standing infection with hepatitis B or C.

SYMPTOMS

Hepatitis B infection rarely shows any symptoms. When it does, the symptoms mimic an acute flu, with fevers, nausea, vomiting, jaundice, abdominal pains, diarrhea, and weight loss.

Hepatitis B can also appear as a very sudden, or fulminant, infection, which is capable of destroying the liver within weeks. In other cases, it can start intensely and then transform into a long-standing chronic condition. Patients with chronic hepatitis B can suffer from other immune conditions affecting their joints or kidneys. It has also been recognized that patients with hepatitis B or C tend to suffer from depression.

TREATMENT

Vaccination for hepatitis B has been available since 1982, and it is important to practice prevention by vaccinating all children. If infection occurs, antiviral drugs such as alpha-interferon, lamivudine, and adefovir dipivoxil can be used in various combinations. These drugs eliminate the infection in 60 percent of cases. However, side effects, including abnormal thyroid function and depression, are common.

HEPATITIS B VIRUS (HBV)	
TRANSMISSION	Through infected blood or bodily fluids: mother to child during birth; using a toothbrush or other personal items from an infected person
AFFECTED POPULATIONS	Recipients of contaminated blood products; infants born to infected mothers; hemodialysis patients; IV drug users; sex contacts of infected persons
PRESENTATION	Either no symptoms or symptoms similar to flu: fever, nausea, vomiting, jaundice, and abdominal pain; diarrhea, weight loss, and dehydration
CHRONIC?	Chronic infection occurs in 90 percent of infants infected at birth, 30 percent of children infected between one and five years of age, and 6 percent in those infected after five years of age
TREATMENT	Vaccination for all children available since 1982. Alpha-interferon, lamivudine, and adefovir dipivoxil are licensed for chronic HBV infection.

HEPATITIS C

Hepatitis C is a major cause of chronic liver disease in many parts of the world, including the United States. No vaccine is available, making hepatitis C the number-one risk factor for cirrhosis and liver cancer. Much research is currently under way to remedy this important problem. In the United States, hepatitis C is commonly seen in children adopted from countries where the blood supply or hospital care were substandard. Sharing needles or receiving tainted blood products is the most common route of transmission, however. (In children, transmission from an infected mother to her infant at birth is also a common route.)

SYMPTOMS

Hepatitis C is a silent infection in more than 80 percent of cases. When the virus is contracted, for example, through a tainted transfusion, it looks like a typical flu, with malaise, fever, shaking chills, nausea, abdominal pain, and fatigue. (Remember though that accurate screening tests for blood transfusions have been in place since 1992 and the likelihood of becoming infected with viral hepatitis via a transfusion is markedly diminished.)

DIAGNOSIS

Diagnosis of hepatitis C infection is confirmed by blood tests revealing antibodies against the virus in the blood. Tests can also identify the virus itself and measure its concentration in the blood. These tests provide important information that will guide treatment.

TREATMENT

To date, there is no vaccine to prevent hepatitis C. The most current and widely used antiviral drugs are interferon and ribavirin, which are used in various combinations. These drugs can eliminate the infection in 60 to 80 percent of cases, depending on the genetic makeup of the virus. However, side effects, including depression, are common.

HEPATITIS C (HCV)	
TRANSMISSION	Through infected blood or bodily fluids; mother to child; shared needles, toothbrush, or other personal items
AFFECTED POPULATIONS	Includes children of infected mothers, those receiving tainted blood products, IV drug users
PRESENTATION	Mostly symptomless; flulike symptoms when acute: fever, chills, aches, nausea, abdominal pain, and fatigue
CHRONIC?	Chronic in 75 to 85 percent of cases; liver disease results in 70 percent of those patients
TREATMENT	Management with drug protocols including interferon and ribavirin

Much progress is being made against viral hepatitis through careful screening of the blood supplies and by public health campaigns aimed at ameliorating the hygienic conditions that increase the risk factors for transmission of the viruses. Moreover, immunization campaigns against hepatitis A and hepatitis B have been very effective in reducing the incidence of these problems in children, especially in those infants who would have contracted hepatitis B from their mothers at birth.

Afterword

When parents take their newborn baby home, they embark on an exciting, rewarding, and challenging new life. Nothing is quite the same once they shoulder this new set of responsibilities; many will look back longingly at lazy weekend hours spent without a care in the world. A new reality dramatically introduces itself as soon as the first breast-feeding is offered or the first diaper is changed. There are surprises around every corner. Bewilderment, anxiety, and panic are totally natural reactions for parents faced with unexpected responses from their baby.

Even the trivial aspects of care can seem daunting when a child appears in distress or is not behaving as expected. Nothing better prepares a parent to tackle this seemingly unending stream of possible sources of stress, however, than information, and information and a sense of perspective is what we aimed to provide in *My Tummy Hurts*.

A well-informed parent is better prepared to figure out possible reasons for his or her child's distress. No one can be expected to know instinctively what is going on! In many cases, anticipating the consequences of an infection or understanding the functioning of the various parts of the digestive tract will help you to prevent or minimize medical problems. There is nothing mysterious about gas, spitting up, or abdominal pain. I hope *My Tummy Hurts* has fulfilled this goal of giving you the confidence to accept digestive problems as manageable. An organized approach based on understanding how it all works will help you face a problem with a clearer head that tells you, above all, that there's no need to panic.

This book also offered advice about how a parent can best approach the common complaint of stomachache and the steps that can be taken to get to the bottom of the problem. The importance of proper nutrition and the effects of various food components in triggering pain, gas, or diarrhea were explored in the hope of expanding your parental arsenal.

Fostering a sense of empowerment through knowledge and confidence is what *My Tummy Hurts* is all about. I hope this book will serve you well throughout your child's development.

Appendix

This list will provide you with additional selected sources and links for most of the topics discussed in this book. Although not comprehensive, these references will still complement pertinent chapters in *My Tummy Hurts*.

North American Society for Pediatric Gastroenterology,
    Hepatology and Nutrition (NASPGHN)
P.O. Box 6
Flourtown, PA 19031
(215) 233-0808
Web site: http://www.naspgn.org

The Web site of the North American Society for Pediatric Gastroenterology, Hepatology and Nutrition offers a wealth of authoritative information and useful links. Among the conditions referenced are anorectal malformations, celiac disease, cyclic vomiting syndrome, gastroesophageal reflux, food allergies, Crohn's disease and colitis, pancreatitis, liver diseases, and motility disorders.

The Children's Hospital of New York-Presbyterian
3959 Broadway
New York, NY 10032

(212) 305-2500

Web site: http://www.childrensnyp.org

The Children's Hospital of New York-Presbyterian, an institution with a long tradition of devotion to children's health care delivery, education, and research, is a great resource for additional information on many of the topics in this book. From their Web site, choose "Child Health A to Z" from the main menu to type your questions.

The National Digestive Diseases Information Clearinghouse (NDDIC)
2 Information Way
Bethesda, MD 20892-3570
(800) 891-5389
E-mail: nddic@info.nddk.nih.gov
Web site for celiac disease:
　　http://www.niddk.nih.gov/health/digest/pubs/celiac/
　　index.htm
Web sites for cyclic vomiting syndrome (CVS):
　　http://www.digestive.niddk.nih.gov/diseases/pubs/cvs/
　　index.htm
　　http://cvsaonline.org
Web site for information on pancreatitis and other pancreatic disorders: http://digestive.niddk.nih.gov/
　　ddiseases/pubs/pancreatitis/index.htm

The National Institutes of Health (NIH)
9000 Rockville Pike
Bethesda, Maryland 20892
Web site for anorexia nervosa and other eating disorders:
　　http://www.nlm.nih.gov/medlineplus/eatingdisorders.html

Web site for the National Institutes of Health's National Center
    for Complementary and Alternative Medicine (NCCAM):
    http://nccam.nih.gov/
Web site for shaken-baby syndrome:
    www.ninds.nih.gov/health__and__medical/disorders/
    shakenbaby.htm

Crohn's and Colitis Foundation of America
386 Park Avenue South, 17th Floor
New York, NY 10016-8804
(800) 932-2423
Web site: http://ccfa.org

Centers for Disease Control and Prevention (CDC)
1600 Clifton Road
Atlanta, GA 30333
(404) 639-3534
(800) 311-3435
Web site for hepatitis, traveler's diarrhea, infectious diarrhea,
    and parasites: http://www.cdc.gov/

National Foundation for Infectious Diseases (NFID)
4733 Bethesda Avenue, Suite 750
Bethesda, MD 20814
(301) 656-0003
Fax: (301) 907-0878
E-mail: info@nfid.org

American Association for the Study of Liver Disease (AASLD)
1729 King Street, Suite 200
Alexandria, VA 22314
(703) 299-9766

Fax: (703) 299-9622
Web site: http://www.aasld.org

American Liver Foundation
75 Maiden Lane, Suite 603
New York, NY 10038
(800) 465-4837
(888) 443-7872
(212) 668-1000
Fax: (212) 483-8179
E-mail: info@liverfoundation.org

Hepatitis Foundation International (HFI)
504 Blick Drive
Silver Spring; MD 20904-2901
(800) 891-0707
(301) 622-4200
Fax: (301) 622-4702
E-mail: hepfi@hepfi.org
Web site: www.hepfi.org

Glossary

Note: Trade names are used for identification purposes only and do not imply endorsement by the author.

A

Achalasia: failure of the lower esophageal sphincter to relax

Acidophilus: Lactobacillus acidophillus, one type of "good" (probiotic) bacteria found in the colon

Acute: of sudden onset (as for pain)

Adenoids: lymphatic tissue at the back of the throat

Adhesions: strands of tissue that grow between the abdominal wall and the intestine or between the loops of intestine, usually after abdominal surgery; can cause blockage

Adrenal glands: glands located on top of the kidneys that secrete adrenaline, among other hormones

Aerophagia: the tendency to swallow air

Alginic acid: a mild antacid that coats and protects the esophagus; it is a component of the over-the-counter antacid Gaviscon

Alpha-1 antitrypsin: a protease inhibitor, or enzyme responsible for inhibiting the breakdown of proteins

Alpha-1-antitrypsin deficiency: a genetically inherited lack of alpha-1 antitrypsin that results in liver disease in newborns or lung emphysema in adults

ALTE (apparent life-threatening event): a frightening episode in which
   a baby experiences changes in skin color, loss of muscle tone, and
   disruptions in heart rate and respiration

Amylase: a pancreatic enzyme responsible for the digestion of starches

Analgesic: pain medication

Anal stenosis: narrowing of the anus

Anemia: low red blood cell count in the circulation

Antibiotic: medication that inhibits or destroys bacteria or parasites;
   amoxicillin, clarithromycin (Biaxin), metronidazole (Flagyl), and
   tetracycline are all examples

Antibody: specific immunoglobulin protein produced in response to an
   infection

Anticonvulsant: drug used to control convulsions (seizures);
   gabapentin phenobarbital (Neurontin) and carbamazepine
   (Tegretol) are examples

Antihypertensive: drug to control high blood pressure; clonidine
   (Catapres) is an example

Antiviral: drug to inhibit the growth of viruses; interferon, ribavirin,
   and lamivudine are examples

Antro-duodenal manometry: test of stomach and duodenum motility

Antrum: the lower, tapered part of the stomach

Anus: the terminal orifice of the intestinal tract

Appendectomy: operation to remove the appendix

Appendicitis: inflammation of the appendix

Appendix: wormlike appendage of intestine opening into the cecum,
   the beginning of the ascending colon

Ascending colon: the first part of the large intestine, or large bowel

Aspiration: penetration of saliva, formula, or food into the lungs

Atherosclerosis: hardening of the arteries

B

Bacteria: plural of bacterium

Bacterium: single-celled organism

Barium: a component of contrast suspensions used for imaging in radiology

Barium enema: a barium suspension introduced through the rectum, used for visualizing the large intestine with X-rays

Barium swallow: diagnostic study of the mechanics of swallowing and examination of the esophagus and stomach with X-rays and an orally ingested barium suspension

Bile: fluid secreted by the liver containing bile acids, cholesterol, and emulsifiers needed for the digestion and absorption of fats

Biliary atresia: congenital complete closure of the bile ducts draining bile from the liver into the duodenum

Bilirubin: the pigment that gives bile its typical green color, derived from the breakdown of old red blood cells in the spleen; it appears yellow in the skin

Biofeedback: behavior-modification technique capable of modifying automatic bodily functions such as blood pressure and heart rate; also used as a coping response to chronic pain or nausea

Biopsy: obtaining a tissue sample for diagnosis

Bisacodyl: a commonly used stimulant laxative; active ingredient of over-the-counter Dulcolax

Body mass index (BMI): a measurement of the degree to which a person is overweight or obese, calculated as the weight/height^2 (BMIs above 25 denote overweight)

Bolus: soft mass of food and saliva ready for swallowing

Bronchi: plural of bronchus

Bronchioles: smallest airways in the respiratory tree

Bronchiolitis: inflammation of the bronchioles

Bronchitis: inflammation of the bronchi

Bronchus: larger air passages of the lungs

C

CAT (computerized axial tomography), or CT, scan: a widely used imaging technique that forms composite images of the body after obtaining multiple cross-sectional X-ray images

Caustic ingestion: drinking products containing strong alkali (such as sodium hydroxide) or acids (such as sulfuric acid); extremely damaging to the lining of the esophagus

CDC: Centers for Disease Control and Prevention, a United States federal agency in charge of protecting the health and safety of its citizens

Cecum: the beginning of the ascending colon

Celiac disease (also called gluten-sensitive enteropathy or non-tropical sprue): a permanent condition resulting from immune-mediated damage to the small intestine caused by exposure to wheat, barley, rye, and oats; can also affect the skin, resulting in dermatitis herpetiformis

Cerebral palsy (CP): nonprogressive brain disorder that affects muscle tone and control of body movements

Choanal atresia: complete obstruction of the nasal passage; can be one-sided or affect both sides, causing breathing and feeding difficulties in the newborn

Cholecystokinin (CCK): hormone involved in the regulation of gallbladder contraction and the sensation of fullness after eating

Cholesterol: one of the important lipids (fats) in the body, a component of all cell membranes and found in high concentrations in the brain; deposits of cholesterol in the wall of arteries results in atherosclerosis

Chronic: persists over a long period

Cirrhosis: scarring of the liver

Clotting factor: protein involved in normal clotting of the blood

Colectomy: complete removal of the colon

Colic, infantile: inconsolable crying and fussiness in an infant, lasting over three hours a day and occurring at least three times a week for over three weeks; typically appearing after three weeks of age, it tends to subside after three months of age

Colitis: inflammation of the colon

Colon: the large intestine

Colonoscopy: direct examination of the inside of the large intestine using an endoscope

Corticotrophin releasing factor (CRF): a brain hormone important in activating the pituitary-to-adrenal axis and part of the body's circadian rhythm; currently believed to play a role in certain cases of cyclic vomiting syndrome

Crohn's disease: chronic immune-mediated inflammation of unknown cause that can involve all portions of the gastrointestinal tract, as well as organs outside of the intestine such as the eyes, joints, skin, and liver

Cryptosporidium: single-cell parasite that affects the gastrointestinal tract causing diarrhea, nausea, and cramps

Cyclic vomiting syndrome (CVS): a condition characterized by repeated episodes of severe, intense vomiting, nausea, and abdominal pains, between which the child is completely normal; often clears by adolescence, when migraines develop in a high proportion of patients

Cytomegalovirus (CMV): a virus responsible for many infections acquired by the developing infant before birth; especially dangerous in patients with impaired immune systems

D

Dermatitis herpetiformis: itchy, hive-like rash caused by an immune reaction to gluten

Diaphragm: the muscles that separate the chest from the abdominal cavity; important in helping the lungs expand and contract during breathing

Dicylomine hydrochloride: drug used to relieve spasm in the digestive tract; found in Bentyl

Distension: overstretching, bloating, or swelling, as of the stomach

Diverticulitis: inflammation of a diverticulum

Duodenum: the first section of the small intestine, which receives food directly from the stomach

Dyschezia: infantile difficulty with passing a bowel movement, caused by immaturity and discoordination of the muscles that expel the stool

Dyspepsia: discomfort, with or without heartburn, centered on the stomach and lower esophagus, usually aggravated by meals

Dysphagia: painful swallowing

Dystonia: imbalance of muscle tone

E

Electrolytes: body salts such as sodium, potassium, and chloride that are needed to keep body fluids balanced properly

Encopresis: passage of stools in inappropriate places, such as in the underpants or on the floor; usually the result of chronic constipation and loss of sphincter control due to chronic stool withholding

Endoscopy: direct view of the inside of the digestive tract using a flexible endoscope; colonoscopy is endoscopy of the colon, gastroscopy is endoscopy of the stomach

Enema: introduction of fluid (medication, barium suspension, laxatives) through the rectum

Enteric nervous system (ENS): the "brain in the gut"; the complex nervous system that controls most intestinal functions, including contractions, blood flow, and sensation

Enterocolitis: inflammation of the small intestine and colon

Enteropathy: a general term used to describe any disease of the intestines

Enzyme: molecule that acts as a catalyst for chemical reactions in the body

Eosinophil: type of white cell that participates in many immune-related allergic reactions in the body

Epigastric: pertaining to the epigastrium, the upper and mid-part of the abdomen, approximately where the ribs join the sternum

Epiglottis: a valve of cartilage that closes over the windpipe to stop food from entering the larynx and penetrating the airway

Epstein–Barr virus (EBV): a cause of mononucleosis

Esophagitis: inflammation of the esophagus

Esophagus: tube of muscle leading from the throat to the stomach

F

Fever: elevated body temperature; physical response to a number of conditions such as infections or inflammation

Fibromyalgia: functional condition with chronic muscle pains and fatigue

Flatus: gas expelled through the anus

Fluoroscopy: X-ray imaging in real time

Fulminant: sudden, devastating, as a disease

Functional pain: a type of pain with no apparent underlying physical cause

Fundus: the upper portion of stomach, which relaxes as food is taken in

G

Gag reflex: automatic closing of the epiglottis triggered by stimulation of the back of the throat

Galactose: one of the simple sugars; a component, with *glucose*, of *lactose*

Galactosemia: congenital metabolic malfunction caused by the inability to process galactose normally

Gallbladder: sac-like organ under surface of the liver on the right upper quadrant of the torso that receives the bile from the liver and stores it until it contracts and expels it into the intestine during a meal

Gallstone: accumulated and enlarged crystals of cholesterol or bilirubin that form in the gallbladder

Gastritis: inflammation of the stomach

Gastrocolic reflex: the automatic activation of colon contractions that promote a bowel movement, triggered by the presence of food in the stomach

Gastroenteritis: inflammation of the lining of the stomach and intestines

Gastrointestinal: pertaining to the digestive system

Gastroschisis: congenital defect in which the abdominal wall is incompletely closed

Gastrostomy: a surgically created opening from the abdominal wall into the stomach through which food can be delivered

GER: gastroesophageal reflux

GERD: gastroesophageal reflux disease

Ghrelin: hormone that signals satiety, or the sensation of fullness, when eating

Giardia lamblia: a common intestinal parasite responsible for diarrhea and abdominal pain

Gliadin: protein component of the gluten in wheat, rye, barley, and possibly oats that stimulates an immune-system response that causes the damage in patients with celiac disease

Glucagon: hormone produced by the pancreas that helps increase glucose levels in the blood

Glucose: a simple sugar needed to provide energy for most body functions; its level in the blood is regulated by insulin

Gluten: component of wheat, rye, barley, and possibly oats that instigates celiac disease

Gluten-sensitive enteropathy: also known as celiac disease, an immune-mediated condition resulting in damage to the intestine and other organs after exposure to gluten

Glycemic index: the degree that a given carbohydrate-containing food can raise the blood levels of glucose in the two hours following its ingestion; possibly an effective indicator of the capacity of foods to promote obesity

Glycemic load: calculated as the glycemic index multiplied by the grams of carbohydrates in a serving size

Glycerol: the water-soluble backbone to which fatty acids are attached in triglyceride fats

Gonads: sex organs—the testicles or ovaries

Granuloma: a collection of large cells typically seen under the microscopic examination of the inflamed tissues of patients with Crohn's disease and also in certain infections like tuberculosis

H

H-2 blocker: drug that inhibits acid production in the stomach by blocking the histamine-2 signal; products such as Zantac and Pepcid are examples

HBIG: hepatitis B immunoglobulin

Henoch-Schönlein purpura: vasculitis, or inflammation of the small arteries, resulting in small hemorrhages in the skin, but can also affect the intestines, joints, and kidneys

Hepatic: pertaining to the liver

Hepatitis B immunoglobulin: immunoglobulin with high concentration of antibodies against hepatitis B, used to protect the newborn exposed to the virus at birth until the vaccine has a chance to work

Hereditary fructose intolerance: congenital metabolic malfunction caused by the inability to process fructose

Hernia: protrusion of tissue or part of an organ through an opening in the cavity that encloses it, such as intestine coming through the groin or the belly button

Herniorrhaphy: operation to repair a hernia

Hiatal hernia: protrusion that occurs when part of the stomach slides into the chest through the hiatal opening of the diaphragm

Hirschsprung's disease: a congenital lack of ganglion cells in the colon that causes intestinal obstruction or chronic constipation.

H. pylori: the bacterium *Helicobacter pylori*

Hormone: chemical delivered through the bloodstream as needed to perform specific bodily functions, such as the control of glucose levels by insulin, a hormone produced in the pancreas

Hyperglycemia: high level of glucose in the blood

Hypersensitivity: excessive response to a stimulus

Hypertension: high blood pressure

Hypertympanic: sounding like a drum

Hypoallergenic: unlikely to trigger an allergic reaction; usually describes a food or other product

Hypogastric: located below the stomach

Hypoglycemia: low level of glucose in the blood

Hypotonia: low muscle tone

I

IBD: inflammatory bowel disease

IBS: irritable bowel syndrome

Idiopathic: of unknown cause

Ileum: last section of the small intestine

Immunodeficiency: a defect in the body's natural defenses against infection

Immunoglobulins: antibody proteins produced in the body in response to infections and foreign substances

Immunosuppression: the state of impaired immunity; can be congenital or secondary to medications given specifically to keep the immune system in check

Inflammatory bowel disease (IBD): a general term given to chronic inflammation of the intestine not caused by a known infection or other identifiable cause; includes ulcerative colitis and Crohn's disease

Insulin: hormone produced in the pancreas responsible for regulating glucose concentrations in the blood

Intussusception: the telescoping of the intestine into itself

Irritable bowel syndrome (IBS): a chronic functional gastrointestinal condition characterized by, among other symptoms, abnormal defecation patterns, pain, and bloatedness

Ischemia: lack of blood supply and oxygen to the tissue

J

Jejunum: the section of the small intestine between the duodenum and the ileum

K

KUB: for "kidneys-ureters-bladder," a commonly obtained abdominal X-ray film; also called a "flat plate"

L

Lactase: the enzyme that breaks down lactose into glucose and galactose

Lactose: the sugar found in milk and milk products

Lactose breath test: diagnostic test for lactose intolerance that measures hydrogen concentrations in exhaled breath after a loading dose of lactose is administered orally

Lactose intolerance: symptoms such as abdominal pain, gassiness, and diarrhea resulting from insufficient activity of the lactase enzyme

Laparoscopy: surgical procedure performed by the introduction of instruments through small incisions

Large intestine: the colon

Larynx: the portion of the back of the throat leading to the vocal chords

Lecithin: agent in bile that keeps fatty cholesterol in a dissolved state

Leptin: hormone that helps regulate body weight and metabolism

Ligament of Treitz: the anchor of the intestine on the back wall of the peritoneum; it is normally located on the left upper quadrant

Lipase: the enzyme produced by the pancreas needed for digestion of fats

M

Malabsorption: impaired absorption of nutrients by the intestine

Malrotation: a type of intestinal obstruction caused by abnormal development of the gut in the fetus

Manometry: measurement of the pressure generated by the contractions of the intestine during peristalsis

Meckel's diverticulum: remnant of the small bowel that connected the fetal intestine to the umbilicus

Mediastinum: the space between the lungs in the middle of the chest

Melena: dark, tarry or sticky stool resulting from an upper-gastrointestinal bleed

Metabolism: the complex chemical reactions responsible for keeping a living organism functioning normally

Methane: hydrocarbon gas produced in the colon by bacteria

Midgut: middle part of the intestine extending from the second portion of the duodenum to the mid-colon

MMR: measles, mumps, rubella vaccine

Modified barium swallow: barium swallow with special attention to the phases of swallowing; performed during the evaluation of feeding difficulties or dysphagia

Modulation: reprocessing of a pain signal as it travels neural pathways

Mononucleosis: an infection caused by the Epstein-Barr virus, or EBV

Motility: the muscle contractions of the esophagus, stomach, duodenum, or colon that produce the coordinated propulsion of food through the digestive tract

Motility studies: tests measuring the strength and timing of the muscle contractions of the esophagus, stomach, duodenum, or colon

MRI (magnetic resonance imaging) test: imaging technique based on the changes caused to body cells and fluids when exposed to a powerful magnet; does not involve radiation exposure

Multiple organ failure: progressive failure of lungs, heart, kidney, and liver as a result of shock

Muscle tone: the resting tension of a muscle

Mycobacteria: infectious agents that cause certain serious infections like tuberculosis

N

Necrotizing enterocolitis: inflammation causing severe injury to bowel (*necrosis* means "death of tissue") occurring in premature infants; believed to be caused by bacterial contamination, immaturity of the bowel immune system, and other factors

NSAIDs: nonsteroidal anti-inflammatory drugs, like ibuprofen and aspirin

O

Omphalocele: congenital condition in which the intestine and other organs are trapped in the umbilical sac

Ondansetron: a commonly used antinausea medication; marketed as Zofran

ORS (oral rehydration solution): a solution of glucose and electrolytes suitable for correction of dehydration caused by diarrheal illnesses

Osteoarthritis: inflammation of the joints

Osteoporosis: a condition in which low bone mass causes thin, fragile bones

OTC (ornithine transcarbamylase) deficiency: a congenital metabolic malfunction characterized by a breakdown in the ability to rid the body of ammonia

P

PADS (persistent abdominal pain syndrome with social disability): a form of functional abdominal pain in children characterized by chronic pain, nausea, dizziness, headaches, and other complaints severe enough to interfere with normal activities and school attendance

Pancreas: organ that produces the enzymes needed to digest food, and insulin and glucagon, the hormones needed to regulate glucose levels

Pancreatitis: inflammation of the pancreas

Pathological: causing disease or contrary to the body's normal function

Peptic ulcer: ulcer caused by acid damage to the wall of the stomach or duodenum

Peristalsis: coordinated sweeping muscular waves that move food through the digestive tract

Peritoneum: the membrane lining the cavity of the abdomen

Peritonitis: inflammation of the peritoneum, the membrane covering all of the intestinal organs

Periumbilical: located around the belly button

Pharynx: the back of the throat

Phototherapy: the treatment of infant jaundice by exposure to light

pH probe study: a diagnostic test for measuring the pattern of acid exposure of the esophagus

Physiological: consistent with the body's normal functioning

Pinworms: Enterobius vermicularis, a small intestinal parasite, causing rectal itching

Pituitary gland: endocrine (hormone producing) gland at the base of the brain that plays a major role in regulating metabolism

Plexus: a network, as of nerves or veins

Polyethylene glycol (PEG): the active component of nonhabit-forming laxatives such as MiraLax

Portal vein: the vein that feeds the liver, created by the convergence of the vein from the intestines and the vein from the spleen

Projectile vomiting: the violent regurgitation of stomach contents

Prokinetics: medications to improve forward peristalsis, an example being cisapride

Proton pump inhibitors (PPIs): antacid drugs that inhibit the transfer of hydrogen (proton) into hydrochloric acid; products such as Prevacid, Prilosec, Nexium, and Protonix are all examples

Psychogenic: originating in the mind

Psyllium: fleawort plant, the husk of which is used in fiber supplements such as Metamucil

Pyloric stenosis: a narrowing of the pyloric channel

Pylorus: the valvelike sphincter between the stomach and the duodenum

R

Raffinose: complex sugar present in beans, lentils, peas

RAP: recurrent abdominal pain

Rectal exam: physical diagnostic examination of the anus and rectum

Rectum: last part of the colon; joins the sigmoid colon to the anus

Remicade: brand name for infliximab, an antibody against TNF-alpha
(tumor necrosis factor alpha), one of the primary molecules that
causes inflammation

Rome II: the diagnostic criteria for functional gastrointestinal
disorders published in 2000

S

Saliva: the fluid secretion produced by glands in the mouth that helps
lubricate and prepare food for swallowing; also contains enzymes
such as amylase and lipase that begin the digestive process

SBS: short bowel syndrome, a malabsorption syndrome resulting from
significant loss of the small intestine

Senna: a plant-derived stimulant laxative; used in Senokot

Sigmoid colon: S-shaped portion of the large intestine following the
descending colon and before the rectum

Sigmoidoscopy: direct examination of the sigmoid colon performed
with an endoscope

Simethicone: active ingredient of gas-relieving preparations such as
Mylicon

SMA: superior mesenteric artery, the main blood vessel supplying the
digestive organs

Small bowel: the small intestine

Small bowel follow-through: diagnostic X-ray test that enables the
examination of the stomach and the entire small bowel until it
reaches the cecum

Small intestine: the section of intestine between the stomach and colon; also called small bowel

Sorbitol: sugar found in fruit like apples, pears, peaches, and prunes; also used as an artificial sweetener in some dietetic products

Spasm: strong, painful muscle contractions

Sphincterotomy: procedure to enlarge the opening of the pancreatic and biliary duct as it drains into the duodenum

Spina bifida: congenital spinal defect

Spleen: an organ closely related to the liver (see *Portal vein*) and responsible for, among other functions, filtering the blood to remove old red blood cells, a process in which bilirubin is formed

SSRI (selective serotonin reuptake inhibitor): a class of antidepressants such as fluoxetine (Prozac) and paroxetine (Paxil) frequently used as pain modulators in chronic functional pains

Stachyose: complex sugar present in beans, lentils, and peas

Steroid: a fat-soluble compound produced by the adrenal glands or the gonads; sex hormones and anti-inflammatory medications such as prednisone, prednisolone, and hydrocortisone are all steroids

Stomach: the muscular baglike organ that receives the food from the esophagus and prepares it for delivery to the duodenum

Stool: feces

Stricture: fixed narrowing in tubes such as the esophagus, bile ducts, or intestine

Substance P: a substance that carries signals in the brain (neurotransmitter) involved in pain perception and nausea

Sulfasalazine: an anti-inflammatory drug used in the management of IBD

Syndrome: a group of symptoms characteristic of a particular illness

T

TE fistula: an abnormal tunnel-like tissue connection between the esophagus and the trachea

Tenesmus: a painful sensation after a bowel movement is complete, in which the need to continue passing stool is still perceived

Terminal ileum: the last segment of the small intestine; separated from the cecum by the ileocecal valve.

Thoracic: pertaining to the chest

Thyroid: a gland in the neck that secretes thyroxin, an important hormone that controls metabolism

Tonsils: lymph nodes in the throat, part of the immune defense system

TPN (total parenteral nutrition): complete intravenous nutrition administered through a large (central) vein

Trachea: the airway, or windpipe

Transverse colon: section of the large intestine running between the ascending colon on the right and the descending colon on the left

Tricyclic antidepressant: a class of antidepressant drug; amitriptyline (Elavil) is an example

Triglyceride: a type of fat composed of glycerol and fatty acids

Triticale: hybrid of wheat and rye

U

Ulcerative colitis: a chronic inflammation of the lining of the large intestine caused by an abnormal immune response in a predisposed individual; of unknown cause

Ulcerative proctitis: inflammation of the lining of the rectum

Ulcerative rectosigmoiditis: inflammation of the lining of the rectum and the sigmoid colon

Ultrasound: diagnostic imaging using high-frequency sound waves

Umbilical hernia: protrusion of a piece of intestine through the umbilicus (belly button)

Umbilicus: the belly button

Universal colitis: an inflammation of the whole colon; also called pancolitis

Upper GI series: diagnostic X-ray study of the esophagus, stomach, and beginning of the small intestine

Urea breath test: diagnostic test for *H. pylori* based on the measurement of labeled carbon dioxide in exhaled breath after a urea load is administered orally

Ureter: tube that drains the urine from the kidney into the bladder

V

Vagus nerve: the most important channel conveying information to the brain from the gut and vice versa; also provides the nerve supply to the heart, affecting its rhythm

Villi: the fingerlike projections that vastly expand the absorptive surface of the lining of the intestine

Volvulus: portion of intestine that has twisted and strangulated its blood supply

X

X-ray: short-wavelength electromagnetic radiation used for diagnostic imaging

Z

Zofran: trade name for ondansetron, a commonly used antinausea medication

Index